EVIDENCE–BASED TREATMENT PLANNING FOR EATING DISORDERS AND OBESITY

EVIDENCE-BASED TREATMENT PLANNING FOR EATING DISORDERS AND OBESITY

DVD COMPANION WORKBOOK

ARTHUR E. JONGSMA, JR.
AND
TIMOTHY J. BRUCE

WILEY

John Wiley & Sons, Inc.

Published by John Wiley & Sons, Inc., Hoboken, New Jersey.
Published simultaneously in Canada.

No part of this publication may be reproduced, stored in a retrieval system, or transmitted in any form or by any means, electronic, mechanical, photocopying, recording, scanning, or otherwise, except as permitted under Section 107 or 108 of the 1976 United States Copyright Act, without either the prior written permission of the Publisher, or authorization through payment of the appropriate per-copy fee to the Copyright Clearance Center, Inc., 222 Rosewood Drive, Danvers, MA 01923, (978) 750-8400, fax (978) 646-8600, or on the web at www.copyright.com. Requests to the Publisher for permission should be addressed to the Permissions Department, John Wiley & Sons, Inc., 111 River Street, Hoboken, NJ 07030, (201) 748-6011, fax (201) 748-6008.

Limit of Liability/Disclaimer of Warranty: While the publisher and author have used their best efforts in preparing this book, they make no representations or warranties with respect to the accuracy or completeness of the contents of this book and specifically disclaim any implied warranties of merchantability or fitness for a particular purpose. No warranty may be created or extended by sales representatives or written sales materials. The advice and strategies contained herein may not be suitable for your situation. You should consult with a professional where appropriate. Neither the publisher nor author shall be liable for any loss of profit or any other commercial damages, including but not limited to special, incidental, consequential, or other damages.

This publication is designed to provide accurate and authoritative information in regard to the subject matter covered. It is sold with the understanding that the publisher is not engaged in rendering professional services. If legal, accounting, medical, psychological or any other expert assistance is required, the services of a competent professional person should be sought.

Designations used by companies to distinguish their products are often claimed as trademarks. In all instances where John Wiley & Sons, Inc. is aware of a claim, the product names appear in initial capital or all capital letters. Readers, however, should contact the appropriate companies for more complete information regarding trademarks and registration.

For general information on our other products and services please contact our Customer Care Department within the United States at (800) 762-2974, outside the United States at (317) 572-3993 or fax (317) 572-4002.

Wiley publishes in a variety of print and electronic formats and by print-on-demand. Some material included with standard print versions of this book may not be included in e-books or in print-on-demand. If this book refers to media such as a CD or DVD that is not included in the version you purchased, you may download this material at http://booksupport.wiley.com. For more information about Wiley products, visit www.wiley.com.

ISBN: 978-0-470-56861-3

Printed in the United States of America

10 9 8 7 6 5 4 3 2 1

Contents

Introduction

This *Workbook* is a companion to the *Evidence-Based Treatment Planning for the Eating Disorders and Obesity DVD*, which is focused on informing mental health therapists, addiction counselors, and students in these fields about evidence-based psychological treatment planning.

Organization

In this *Workbook* you will find in each chapter:

➤ Summary highlights of content shown in the DVD
➤ Chapter review discussion questions
➤ Chapter review test questions
➤ Chapter references
➤ Key points for review

In appropriate chapters, the references are divided into those for *empirical support,* those for *clinical resources,* and those for *bibliotherapy resources*. Empirical Support references are selected studies or reviews of the empirical work supporting the efficacy of the empirically supported treatments (ESTs) discussed in the chapter. The clinical resources are books, manuals, or other resources for clinicians that describe the application, or "how to," of the treatments discussed. The Bibliotherapy Resources are selected publications and Web sites relevant to the DVD content that may be helpful to clinicians, clients, or laypersons.

Examples of client homework are included at www.wiley.com/go/edowb. They are designed to enhance understanding of therapeutic interventions, in addition to being potentially useful clinically.

Appendix A contains an example of an evidence-based treatment plan for Anorexia Nervosa. In Appendix B, correct and incorrect answers to all chapter review test questions are explained.

Chapter Points

This DVD is electronically marked with chapter points that delineate the beginning of discussion sections throughout the program. You may skip to any one of these chapter points on the DVD by clicking on the forward arrow. The chapter points for this program are as follows:

> ➤ Defining Eating Disorders and Obesity
> ➤ Six Steps in Building a Psychotherapy Treatment Plan
> ➤ Brief History of the EST Movement
> ➤ ESTs for Eating Disorders and Obesity
> ➤ Integrating ESTs for Eating Disorders and Obesity Into a Treatment Plan
> ➤ Common Considerations in Relapse Prevention
> ➤ An Evidence-Based Treatment Plan for Anorexia Nervosa

Series Rationale

Evidence-based practice (EBP) is steadily becoming the standard of mental health care as it has in medical health care. Borrowing from the Institute of Medicine's definition (Institute of Medicine, 2001), the American Psychological Association (APA) has defined EBP as "the integration of the best available research with clinical expertise in the context of patient characteristics, culture, and preferences" (American Psychological Association Presidential Task Force on Evidence-Based Practice (APA), 2006).

Professional organizations such as the American Psychological Association, the National Association of Social Workers, and the American Psychiatric Association, as well as consumer organizations such the National Alliance for the Mentally Ill (NAMI), are endorsing EBP. At the federal level, a major joint initiative of the National Institute of Mental Health and Department of Health and Human Services' Substance Abuse and Mental Health Services Administration (SAMHSA) focuses on promoting, implementing, and evaluating evidence-based mental health programs and practices within state mental health systems (APA, 2006). In some practice settings, EBP is even becoming mandated. It is clear that the call for evidence-based practice is being increasingly sounded.

Unfortunately, many mental health care providers cannot or do not stay abreast of results from clinical research and how they can inform their practices. Although it has rightfully been argued that the relevance of some research to the clinician's needs is weak, there are products of clinical research whose efficacy has been well established and whose effectiveness in the community setting has received support. Clinicians and clinicians-in-training interested in empirically informing their treatments could benefit from educational programs that make this goal more easily attainable.

This series of DVDs and companion workbooks is designed to introduce clinicians and students to the process of empirically informing their psychotherapy treatment plans. The series begins with an introduction to the efforts to identify research-supported treatments and how the products of these efforts can be used to inform treatment planning. The other programs in the series focus on empirically informed treatment planning for each of several commonly seen clinical problems. In each problem-focused DVD, issues involved in defining or diagnosing the presenting problem are reviewed. Research-supported treatments for the problem are described, as well as the process used to identify them. Viewers are then systematically guided through the process of creating a treatment plan, and shown how the plan can be informed by goals, objectives, and interventions consistent with those of the identified research-supported treatments. Example vignettes of selected interventions are also provided.

This series is intended to be educational and informative in nature and not meant to be a substitute for clinical training in the specific interventions discussed and demonstrated. References to empirical support of the treatments described, clinical resource material, and training opportunities are provided.

Exhibit I.1   Dr. Tim Bruce and Dr. Art Jongsma

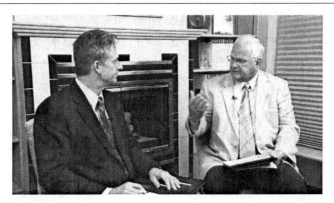

Presenters

Dr. Art Jongsma is the Series Editor and co-author of the Practice*Planners*® series published by John Wiley & Sons. He has authored or co-authored over 40 books in this series. Among the books included in this series are the highly regarded *The Complete Adult Psychotherapy Treatment Planner*, *The Adolescent* and *The Child Psychotherapy Treatment Planners*, and *The Addiction Treatment Planner*. All of these books along with *The Severe and Persistent Mental Illness Treatment Planner*, *The Family Therapy Treatment Planner*, *The Couples Psychotherapy Treatment Planner*, *The Older*

Adult Psychotherapy Treatment Planner, and *The Veterans and Active Duty Military Psychotherapy Treatment Planner* are informed with objectives and interventions that are supported by research evidence.

Dr. Jongsma also created the clinical record management software tool Thera*Scribe*®, which uses point- and- click technology to easily develop, store, and print treatment plans, progress notes, and homework assignments. He has conducted treatment planning and software training workshops for mental health professionals around the world.

Dr. Jongsma's clinical career began as a psychologist in a large private psychiatric hospital. He worked in the hospital for about 10 years and then transitioned to outpatient work in his own private practice clinic, Psychological Consultants, in Grand Rapids, Michigan for 25 years. He has been writing best-selling books and software for mental health professionals since 1995. He lives in a suburb of Grand Rapids with his wife, Judy.

Dr. Timothy Bruce is a Professor and Associate Chair of the Department of Psychiatry and Behavioral Medicine at the University of Illinois, College of Medicine in Peoria, Illinois, where he also directs medical student education. He is a licensed clinical psychologist who completed his graduate training at SUNY-Albany under the mentorship of Dr. David Barlow and his residency training at Wilford Hall Medical Center under the direction of Dr. Robert Klepac. In addition to maintaining an active clinical practice at the university, Dr. Bruce has written numerous publications including books, professional journal articles, book chapters, and professional educational materials, many on the topic of evidence-based practice. Most recently, he has served as the developmental editor empirically informing Dr. Jongsma's best-selling Practice*Planners*® series.

Dr. Bruce is also Executive Director of the Center for the Dissemination of Evidence-based Mental Health Practices, a state- and federally funded initiative to disseminate evidence-based psychological and pharmacological practices across Illinois. Highly recognized as an educator, Dr. Bruce has received nearly thirty awards for his teaching of students and professionals during his career.

References

American Psychological Association Presidential Task Force on Evidence-Based Practice. (2006). Evidence-based practice in psychology. *American Psychologist, 61,* 271–285.

Berghuis, D., Jongsma, A., & Bruce, T. (2006). *The severe and persistent mental illness treatment planner* (2nd ed.). Hoboken, NJ: John Wiley.

Dattilio, F., Jongsma, A., & Davis, S. (2009). *The family therapy treatment planner* (2nd ed.). Hoboken, NJ: John Wiley.

Institute of Medicine. (2001). *Crossing the quality chasm: A new health system for the 21st century*. Washington, DC: National Academy Press.

Jongsma, A., Peterson, M. & Bruce, T. (2006). *The complete adult psychotherapy treatment planner* (4th ed.). Hoboken, NJ: John Wiley.

Jongsma, A., Peterson, M., McInnis, W. & Bruce, T. (2006a). *The adolescent psychotherapy treatment planner* (4th ed.). Hoboken, NJ: John Wiley.

Jongsma, A., Peterson, M., McInnis, W., & Bruce, T. (2006b). *The child psychotherapy treatment planner* (4th ed.). Hoboken, NJ: John Wiley.

Moore, B., & Jongsma, A. (2009). *The veterans and active duty military psychotherapy treatment planner*. Hoboken, NJ: John Wiley.

Perkinson, R., Jongsma, A., & Bruce, T. (2009). *The addiction treatment planner* (4th ed.). Hoboken, NJ: John Wiley.

1

What Are Eating Disorders and Obesity?

Defining Eating Disorders

In this program, we are going to discuss evidence-based treatment planning for eating disorders and obesity. Let's begin by looking at the criteria for eating disorders according to the *Diagnostic and Statistical Manual of Mental Disorders* (DSM). Eating disorders are characterized by clinically significant disturbances in eating behavior. There are two major eating disorders recognized in the *DSM*: Anorexia Nervosa (AN) and Bulimia Nervosa (BN). The essential feature of AN is a refusal to maintain a minimally normal body weight. BN is characterized by repeated episodes of binge eating, as well as problematic compensatory behaviors aimed at preventing weight gain. Binging is defined as the uncontrolled consumption of abnormally large amounts of food in a discrete period. Examples of compensatory behaviors aimed at preventing weight gain include purging the body of the food through self-induced vomiting or misuse of laxatives, diuretics, enemas, or other medications. Fasting and excessive exercise are examples of nonpurging compensatory behaviors.

Long recognized by patients, clinicians, and researchers as a clinically significant eating problem, Binge-Eating Disorder (BED) was not a recognized diagnosis in the *DSM-IV*. It has been proposed as one for the next edition of the manual, *DSM-5*. BED is characterized by frequent episodes of binge eating, but unlike BN, BED is not associated with the compensatory behaviors aimed at preventing weight gain. Consequently, most individuals with BED are overweight, suffer negative emotional consequences as a result of the uncontrolled behavior, and engage in ongoing attempts to diet.

Defining Obesity

Obesity is defined as an excess of body weight, relative to height, that is attributed to an abnormally high proportion of body fat. Because it predisposes individuals to an increased risk of several diseases and medical conditions, obesity is included in the *International Classification of Diseases* (or ICD) as a general medical condition. It does not appear in the *DSM* as an eating disorder because it is not consistently associated with a psychological or behavioral syndrome. It is, however, a highly prevalent medical issue, influenced by psychological and behavioral factors, and has proven to be responsive to psychological treatment. Therefore, we are including obesity in our discussion of psychotherapy treatment planning for eating disorders, although technically speaking it is not an eating disorder.

DSM Diagnostic Criteria for Anorexia Nervosa

Those with AN refuse to maintain a minimally normal body weight, which is defined diagnostically as less than 85% of normal expected weight. Even though they are underweight, people with AN have an intense fear of gaining weight or becoming what they see as fat. Most have a distorted perception of their body shape, seeing it as bigger, heavier, or "fatter" than it is. Many also overvalue body weight and shape in their self-concept, or deny the seriousness of their low body weight. Females with anorexia suffer amenorrhea caused by weight loss, which is defined diagnostically as having missed three consecutive menstrual cycles. Some clients with AN engage in binge eating and purging, whereas others do not. These two subtypes are to be specified when making the diagnosis by indicating whether it is the Binge-eating/Purging Type or the Restricting Type.

The *DSM-IV* Diagnostic Criteria for AN are summarized in Figure 1.1

Figure 1.1

DSM Diagnostic Criteria for Anorexia Nervosa

A. Refusal to maintain body weight at or above a minimally normal weight for age and height
B. Intense fear of gaining weight or becoming fat, even though underweight
C. Disturbance in the way in which one's body weight or shape is experienced, undue influence of body weight or shape on self-evaluation, or denial of the seriousness of the current low body weight
D. In postmenarcheal females, amenorrhea (i.e., the absence of at least three consecutive menstrual cycles)

SPECIFY TYPE:

- Binge-Eating/Purging Type: During the current episode of Anorexia Nervosa, the person has regularly engaged in binge-eating or purging behavior.
- Restricting Type: During the current episode of Anorexia Nervosa, the person has not regularly engaged in binge-eating or purging behavior.

Epidemiology of Anorexia Nervosa

Selected epidemiological information for AN is summarized in Figure 1.2.

Figure 1.2

Anorexia Nervosa Epidemiology

- Lifetime prevalence: .5%
- Gender distribution: 90% female
- Age of onset: 14–18 years
- Long-term mortality: ~10%
- Common causes of death: Starvation, suicide, electrolyte imbalance

---

DSM Diagnostic Criteria for Bulimia Nervosa

The first essential feature of BN is binge eating a large amount of food in which there is a sense of lack of control over the eating. Second, BN is characterized by inappropriate compensatory behaviors to prevent weight gain. For diagnostic purposes, the episodes of binge eating and compensatory behavior should occur, on average, at least twice a week for three months. As with AN, the BN sufferer's self-evaluation is unreasonably influenced by his or her perceived body shape and weight.

Finally, because binging and purging can occur within anorexia nervosa, it is important to rule out that these behaviors are not occurring within the context of that disorder—where body weight is severely compromised and menstrual periods have ceased. The *DSM* asks the diagnostician to distinguish between two subtypes of BN: the Purging Type and the Nonpurging Type. As we have noted, the purging subtype would indicate the use of self-induced vomiting or misuse of laxatives, diuretics, enemas, or other medications to rid the body of food. Nonpurging compensatory behaviors include fasting and excessive exercise.

The *DSM-IV* diagnostic criteria for BN are summarized in Figure 1.3.

Epidemiology of Bulimia Nervosa

Selected epidemiological information for BN is summarized in Figure 1.4.

Criteria for Binge-Eating Disorder

BED is currently not a recognized diagnosis in the *DSM*, but it is proposed as one for the next edition, *DSM-5*. The following are the proposed criteria for the diagnosis, and they reflect its long-recognized clinical features. As its name implies, BED is

Figure 1.3

DSM Diagnostic Criteria for Bulimia Nervosa

A. Recurrent episodes of binge eating. An episode of binge eating is characterized by both of the following:

   (1) Eating, in a discrete period (e.g., within any two-hour period), an amount of food that is definitely larger than most people would eat during a similar period and under similar circumstances.

   (2) A sense of lack of control over eating during the episode (e.g., a feeling that one cannot stop eating or control what or how much one is eating).

B. Recurrent inappropriate compensatory behavior in order to prevent weight gain, such as self-induced vomiting; misuse of laxatives, diuretics, enemas, or other medications; fasting; or excessive exercise.

C. The binge eating and inappropriate compensatory behaviors both occur, on average, at least twice a week for three months.

D. Self-evaluation is unduly influenced by body shape and weight.

E. The disturbance does not occur exclusively during episodes of Anorexia Nervosa.

SPECIFY TYPE:

- Purging Type: During the current episode of Bulimia Nervosa, the person has regularly engaged in self-induced vomiting or the misuse of laxatives, diuretics, or enemas.
- Nonpurging Type: During the current episode of Bulimia Nervosa, the person has used other inappropriate compensatory behaviors, such as fasting or excessive exercise, but has not regularly engaged in self-induced vomiting or the misuse of laxatives, diuretics, or enemas.

Figure 1.4

Bulimia Nervosa Epidemiology

- Lifetime prevalence: 1–3%
- Gender distribution: 90% female
- Average age of onset: 18

characterized by recurrent episodes of binge eating. Binge-eating episodes are often characterized by eating more quickly than usual, eating until uncomfortably full, or eating large amounts of food when not physically hungry. Those with BED often eat alone, out of embarrassment, and they often feel disgusted, depressed, or guilty after a binging episode. BED causes marked distress in the individual, and for diagnostic purposes needs to occur, on average, at least weekly for three months or more. Unlike bulimia, BED is not associated with attempts to counteract the effects of binge eating, such as purging. Consequently, most individuals with this disorder are overweight and engage in ongoing attempts to diet.

The proposed diagnostic criteria for BED are summarized in Figure 1.5.

Figure 1.5

Proposed Diagnostic Criteria for Binge-Eating Disorder

A. Recurrent episodes of binge eating. An episode of binge eating is characterized by both of the following:

   (1) Eating, in a discrete period (for example, within any 2-hour period), an amount of food that is definitely larger than most people would eat in a similar period under similar circumstances

   (2) A sense of lack of control over eating during the episode (for example, a feeling that one cannot stop eating or control what or how much one is eating)

B. The binge-eating episodes are associated with three (or more) of the following:

   (1) Eating much more rapidly than normal

   (2) Eating until feeling uncomfortably full

   (3) Eating large amounts of food when not feeling physically hungry

   (4) Eating alone because of feeling embarrassed by how much one is eating

   (5) Feeling disgusted with oneself, depressed, or very guilty afterward

C. Marked distress regarding binge eating is present.

D. The binge eating occurs, on average, at least once a week for 3 months.

NOTE:

- In BED, there are no compensatory behaviors.
- Most people with BED are overweight.
- There are often multiple attempts at dieting.

Epidemiology of Binge-Eating Disorder

Selected epidemiological information for BED is summarized in Figure 1.6.

Figure 1.6

Binge-Eating Disorder Epidemiology

- Lifetime prevalence: 3.5% females, 2.0% males
- Gender distribution: 60% female, 40% males
- Age of onset: 16–24

Criteria for Obesity

As we have noted, obesity is defined as an excess of body fat, relative to height, that is attributed to an abnormally high proportion of body fat. A common metric used to calculate the presence and degree of obesity is the body mass index (BMI). For adults, a BMI of 25–29.9 is classified as overweight. A BMI over 30 constitutes obesity. While there is no scientifically accepted definition of obesity in children and adolescents, pediatric overweight is typically defined as a BMI-for-age meeting or exceeding the 95th percentile; the 85th percentile marks the point at which a child or adolescent is considered at risk for being overweight.

Overweight and obesity are established risk factors for several medical complications and diseases, including high blood pressure, diabetes, and coronary artery disease. Obesity is not an eating disorder per se, but rather a medical condition. It is, however, strongly influenced by psychological and behavioral factors and has been shown to be responsive to psychological treatment.

The diagnostic criteria for obesity are summarized in Figure 1.7.

Figure 1.7

Diagnostic Criteria for Obesity

An excess of body weight, relative to height, that is attributed to an abnormally high proportion of body fat. Excess defined by BMI:

- Body Mass Index (BMI) Formula: weight in kilograms/height in meters^2 or (weight in lbs./height in inches^2) x 703
- A BMI of 30 or more is considered obese. For children, a BMI-for-age meeting or exceeding the 95th percentile is considered obese.

Epidemiology of Obesity

Selected epidemiological information for obesity is summarized in Figure 1.8.

Figure 1.8

Obesity Epidemiology

- Prevalence by gender is 32% of adult men and 35% of adult women.
- Obesity rate in children ages 2 to 19 is estimated at 17%.

Key Points

- Eating disorders are characterized by clinically significant disturbances in eating behavior.
- The essential feature of AN is a refusal to maintain a minimally normal body weight.
- BN is characterized by repeated episodes of binge eating, as well as problematic compensatory behaviors aimed at preventing weight gain.
  - Binging is defined as the uncontrolled consumption of abnormally large amounts of food in a discrete period.
  - Examples of compensatory behaviors aimed at preventing weight gain include purging the body of food through self-induced vomiting or misuse of laxatives, diuretics, enemas, or other medications. Fasting and excessive exercise are examples of nonpurging compensatory behaviors.
- BED is characterized by frequent episodes of binge eating, but unlike BN, BED is not associated with the compensatory behaviors aimed at preventing weight gain.
- Obesity is not an eating disorder per se, but rather a medical condition. It is, however, strongly influenced by psychological and behavioral factors and has been shown to be responsive to psychological treatment. Obesity is defined as an excess of body weight, relative to height, that is attributed to an abnormally high proportion of body fat.

Chapter Review

1. What are the diagnostic criteria for Anorexia Nervosa?
2. What are the diagnostic criteria for Bulimia Nervosa?
3. What are proposed diagnostic criteria for Binge-Eating Disorder?
4. How is obesity defined medically?

Chapter Review Test Questions

1. Which of the following best differentiates bulimia nervosa (BN) from binge-eating disorder (BED)?

    A. BED is not associated with the compensatory behaviors aimed at preventing weight gain characteristic of BN.
    B. BN is not associated with the binge eating characteristic of BED.
    C. In BED, body weight is significantly lower than normal relative to BN.
    D. There are more attempts to diet in BN than in BED.

2. True or False? Binge eating is characteristic of bulimia nervosa and binge-eating disorder, but is not seen in anorexia nervosa (AN).

References

American Psychiatric Association. (2000). *Diagnostic and statistical manual of mental disorders* (4th ed., text rev.). Washington, DC: American Psychiatric Association.

American Psychiatric Association. DSM-5 Development. At www.dsm5.org

2

What Are the Six Steps in Building a Treatment Plan?

Step 1: Identify primary and secondary problems
> Use evidence-based psychosocial assessment procedures to determine the most significant problem or problems related to current distress, disability, or both.

Step 2: Describe the problem's behavioral manifestations (symptom pattern)
> Note how the problem(s) is evident in your particular client. These features may correspond to the diagnostic criteria for the problem.

Step 3: Make a diagnosis based on *DSM/ICD* criteria
> Based on an evaluation of the client's complete clinical presentation, determine the appropriate diagnosis using the process and criteria described in the *DSM* or the *ICD*.

Step 4: Specify long-term goals
> These goal statements need not be crafted in measurable terms, but are broader and indicate a desired general positive outcome of treatment.

Step 5: Create short-term objectives
> Objectives for the client to achieve should be stated in measurable or observable terms so accountability is enhanced.

Step 6: Select therapeutic interventions
> Interventions are the actions of the clinician within the therapeutic alliance designed to help the client accomplish the treatment objectives. There should be at least one intervention planned for each client objective.

Key Point

One important aspect of effective treatment planning is that each plan should be tailored to the individual client's particular problems and needs. Treatment plans should not be boilerplate, even if clients have similar problems. Consistent with the definition of an evidence-based practice, the individual's strengths and weaknesses, unique stressors, cultural and social network, family circumstances, and symptom patterns must be considered in developing a treatment strategy. Clinicians should rely on their own good clinical judgment and plan a treatment that is appropriate for the distinctive individual with whom they are working.

Chapter Review

1. What are the six steps involved in developing a psychotherapy treatment plan?

Chapter Review Test Questions

1. As noted previously, some patients with eating disorders may use compensatory behaviors aimed at preventing weight gain, and some do not. Those who do may use purging types (e.g., self-induced vomiting), while others may not (e.g., excessive exercise). In which step of treatment planning would you record the particular expressions of the eating disorder for your individual client?

    A. Creating short-term objectives
    B. Describing the problem's manifestations
    C. Identifying the primary problem
    D. Selecting treatment interventions

2. The statement "Learn and implement coping skills to resist urges to purge the body of food (i.e., to surf the urge)" is an example of a statement describing which of the following elements of a psychotherapy treatment plan?

    A. A primary problem
    B. A short-term objective
    C. A symptom manifestation
    D. A treatment intervention

Chapter References

American Psychological Association Presidential Task Force on Evidence-Based Practice. (2006). Evidence-based practice in psychology. *American Psychologist, 61*, 271–185.

Jongsma, A. (2005). Psychotherapy treatment plan writing. In G. P. Koocher, J. C. Norcross, and S. S. Hill (Eds.), *Psychologists' desk reference* (2nd ed., pp. 232–236). New York, NY: Oxford University Press.

Jongsma, A., Peterson, M., & Bruce, T. (2006). *The complete adult psychotherapy treatment planner* (4th ed.). Hoboken, NJ: Wiley.

Jongsma, A., Peterson, M., McInnis, W., & Bruce, T. (2006). *The adolescent psychotherapy treatment planner* (4th ed.). Hoboken, NJ: Wiley.

CHAPTER 3

What Is the Brief History of the Empirically Supported Treatments Movement?

In the United States, the effort to identify empirically supported treatments (ESTs) began with an initiative of the American Psychological Association's Division 12, The Society of Clinical Psychology.

In 1993, APA's Division 12 President David Barlow initiated a task group, chaired by Diane Chambless. The group was charged to review the psychotherapy outcome literature to identify psychological treatments whose efficacy had been demonstrated through clinical research. This group was originally called the Task Force on the Promotion and Dissemination of Psychological Procedures and was later reorganized under the Task Force on Psychological Interventions.

Process Used to Identify ESTs

Reviewers established two primary sets of criteria for judging the evidence base supporting any particular therapy. One was labeled *well-established*, the other *probably efficacious* (Figure 3.1).

Key Point

Division 12's criteria for a well-established treatment are similar to the standards used by the United States Food and Drug Administration (FDA) to evaluate the safety and efficacy of proposed medications. The FDA requires demonstration that a proposed medication is significantly superior to a nonspecific control treatment (a pill placebo) in at least two randomized controlled trials conducted by independent research groups. Division 12's criteria for a well-established treatment require the equivalent of this standard as well as other features relevant to judging a psychological treatment's efficacy (e.g., a clear description of the treatment and study participants). By extension, if the FDA were to evaluate psychotherapies using the criteria they use for medication, it would allow sale of those judged to be well-established.

Figure 3.1

Specific Criteria for Well-Established and Probably Efficacious Treatments

Criteria for a Well-Established Treatment

For a psychological treatment to be considered *well-established*, the evidence base supporting it had to be characterized by the following:

I. At least two good between-group design experiments demonstrating efficacy in one or more of the following ways:

  A. Superior (statistically significantly so) to pill or psychological placebo or to another treatment.

  B. Equivalent to an already established treatment in experiments with adequate sample sizes.

OR

II. A large series of single-case design experiments (n > 9) demonstrating efficacy. These experiments must have:

  A. Used good experimental designs

  B. Compared the intervention to another treatment as in IA

Further Criteria for Both I and II

III. Experiments must be conducted with treatment manuals.

IV. Characteristics of the client samples must be clearly specified.

V. Effects must have been demonstrated by at least two different investigators or investigating teams.

Criteria for a Probably Efficacious Treatment

For a psychological treatment to be considered *probably efficacious*, the evidence base supporting it had to meet the following criteria:

I. Two experiments showing the treatment is superior (statistically significantly so) to a waiting-list control group

OR

II. One or more experiments meeting the Well-Established Treatment Criteria IA or IB, III, and IV, but not V

OR

III. A small series of single-case design experiments (n > 3) otherwise meeting Well-Established Treatment

---

Adapted from "Update on Empirically Validated Therapies, II," by D. L. Chambless, M. J. Baker, D. H. Baucom, L. E. Beutler, K. S. Calhoun, P. Crits-Christoph, . . . S. R. Woody, 1998, *The Clinical Psychologist, 51*(1), 3–16.

Products of EST Reviews

The products of these reviews can be found in the Division 12 groups' final two reports.

➤ In the first report, 47 ESTs are identified (Chambless et al., 1996).
➤ In the final report, the list had grown to 71 ESTs (Chambless et al., 1998).
➤ In 1999, The Society of Clinical Psychology, Division 12, took full ownership of maintaining the growing list. The current list and information center can be found on its Web site at: http://www.psychologicaltreatments.org

Around this same time, other groups emerged, using the same or similar criteria, to review literatures related to other populations, problems, and interventions. These and more recent examples include the following:

➤ Children (Lonigan & Elbert, 1998)
➤ Pediatric Psychology (Spirito, 1999)
➤ Older Adults (Gatz, 1998)
➤ Adult, Child, Marital, Family Therapy (Kendall & Chambless, 1998)
➤ Psychopharmacology and Psychological Treatments (Nathan & Gorman, 1998; 2002; 2007)
➤ Eating Disorders (Hay, 2008)

For those interested in comparing and contrasting the criteria used by various review groups, see Chambless and Ollendick (2001).

TherapyAdvisor

Descriptions of the treatments identified through many of these early reviews, as well as references to the empirical work supporting them, clinical resources, and training opportunities, can be found at www.therapyadvisor.com. This resource was developed by Personal Improvement Computer Systems (PICS) with funding from the National Institute of Mental Health and in consultation with members of the original Division 12 task groups. Information found on TherapyAdvisor is provided by the primary author/researcher(s) of the given EST.

Selected Organizational Reviewers of Evidence–Based Psychological Treatments and Practices

➤ Great Britain was on the forefront of the effort to identify evidence-based treatments and develop guidelines for practice. The latest products of their work can be found on the Web site for the National Institute for Health and Clinical Excellence (NICE): http://www.nice.org.uk/

➤ The Substance Abuse and Mental Health Services Administration (SAMHSA) has an initiative to evaluate, identify, and provide information on various mental health practices. Their work, entitled "The National Registry of Evidence-based Programs and Practices or NREPP," can be found online at http://www.nrepp.samhsa.gov/

➤ The Agency for Health Care Policy and Research, now called the Agency for Healthcare Research and Quality (AHRQ), has established guidelines and criteria for identifying evidence-based practices and provides links to evidence-based clinical practice guidelines for various medical and mental health problems at http://www.ahrq.gov/clinic/epcix.htm

➤ Lastly, the Cochrane Collaboration is an international network of professionals who conduct systematic reviews of research in human health care and health policy. Among their products are critical reviews of psychological treatment interventions and specific intervention questions. They can be found on the Web at www.cochrane.org

Other Reviews

Other reviews can be found in the reference section of Chapter 4 under "Empirical Support."

Chapter Review

1. How did Division 12 of the APA identify ESTs?
2. What are the primary differences between *well-established* and *probably efficacious* criteria used to identify ESTs?
3. Where can information about ESTs and evidence-based practices be found?

Chapter Review Test Questions

1. Which statement best describes the process used to identify ESTs?

   A. Consumers of mental health services nominated therapies.
   B. Experts came to a consensus based on their experiences with the treatments.
   C. Researchers submitted their works.
   D. Task groups reviewed the literature using clearly defined selection criteria for ESTs.

2. Based on the differences in their criteria, in which of the following ways are *well-established* treatments different from those classified as *probably efficacious*?

   A. Only *probably efficacious* allowed the use of single-case design experiments.

    B. Only *well-established* allowed studies comparing the treatment to a psycho-logical placebo.

    C. Only *well-established* required demonstration by at least two different, inde-pendent investigators or investigating teams.

    D. Only *well-established* allowed studies comparing the treatment to a pill placebo.

Chapter References

Chambless, D. L., & Ollendick, T. H. (2001). Empirically supported psychologi-cal interventions: Controversies and evidence. *Annual Review of Psychology, 52,* 685–716.

Chambless, D. L., Sanderson, W. C., Shoham, V., Bennett Johnson, S., Pope, K. S., Crits-Christoph, P., . . . McCurry, S. (1996). An update on empirically validated therapies. *The Clinical Psychologist, 49,* 5–18.

Chambless, D. L., Baker, M. J., Baucom, D. H., Beutler, L. E., Calhoun, K. S., Crits-Christoph, P., . . . Woody, S. R. (1998). Update on empirically validated therapies, II. *The Clinical Psychologist, 51,* 3–16.

Gatz, M., Fiske, A., Fox, L. S., Kaskie, B., Kasl-Godley, J. E., McCallum, T., & Wetherell, J. L. (1998). Empirically validated psychological treatments for older adults. *Journal of Mental Health and Aging, 41,* 9–46.

Hay, P. J. (2008). Eating disorders. In J. A. Trafton & W. Gordon (Eds.), *Best practices in the behavioral management of health from preconception to adolescence.* Los Altos, CA: The Institute for Brain Potential.

Kendall, P. C., & Chambless, D. L. (Eds.). (1998). Empirically supported psychologi-cal therapies [special issue]. *Journal of Consulting and Clinical Psychology, 66*(3), 151–162.

Lonigan, C. J., & Elbert, J. C. (Eds.). (1998). Empirically supported psychosocial interventions for children [special issue]. *Journal of Clinical Child Psychology, 27,* 138–226.

Nathan, P. E., & Gorman, J. M. (Eds.). (1998). *A guide to treatments that work.* New York, NY: Oxford University Press.

Nathan, P. E., & Gorman, J. M. (Eds.). (2002). *A guide to treatments that work* (2nd ed.). New York, NY: Oxford University Press.

Nathan, P. E., & Gorman, J. M. (Eds.). (2007). *A guide to treatments that work* (3rd ed.). New York, NY: Oxford University Press.

Spirito, A. (Ed.). (1999). Empirically supported treatments in pediatric psychology [special issue]. *Journal of Pediatric Psychology, 24,* 87–174.

CHAPTER 4

What Are the Identified Empirically Supported Treatments for Eating Disorders and Obesity?

Empirically informing a treatment plan as described in this series involves integrating those aspects of empirically supported treatments (ESTs) into each step of the treatment planning process that was discussed previously. Let's now look at efforts to develop and identify ESTs and evidence-based treatment guidelines for eating disorders and obesity.

Several independent reviews of the psychotherapy outcome literature for the treatment of eating disorders and obesity have identified either empirically supported treatments or support evidence-based practice guidelines. Examples include APA's Division 12 (The Society of Clinical Psychology) and Division 53 (The Society of Clinical Child and Adolescent Psychology), as well as Wilson and Fairburn in Nathan and Gorman's series "A Guide to Treatments that Work." Other organizational reviews have been conducted by the Agency for Healthcare Research and Quality in the United States, the National Institute for Health and Clinical Excellence (or NICE) in Great Britain, and the American Academy of Pediatrics, for example.

ESTs for Anorexia Nervosa

Despite the clinical significance of anorexia nervosa (AN), the psychotherapy outcome literature and practice guidelines based on it have only recently begun to see the type of high-quality controlled studies needed to support evidence-based recommendations.

Family-Based Treatment

A form of family therapy, referred to as the Maudsley Model, has very recently demonstrated efficacy in high-quality studies of both short- and long-term outcomes. This recent advance in the literature has been recognized by several, more recent reviewers of this literature. For example, Divisions 12 and 53 of the APA have recognized family therapy based on the Maudsley Model as well-established for the treatment of AN. The American Academy of Pediatrics has also endorsed this form of family therapy as the outpatient treatment of choice for the disorder.

Family-Based Treatment (FBT) for AN is an outpatient intervention for adolescents. It is designed to restore and maintain weight without hospitalization. Patients who are medically unstable are hospitalized initially, before being discharged to FBT. FBT is conceptualized in three phases and conducted in approximately 20 sessions over the course of one year, although the length of treatment may vary either way depending on clinical progress.

In the first phase of FBT, the seriousness of the disorder is conveyed. Parents are placed in charge of the nutritional rehabilitation and weight restoration of their adolescent child. The family eats some meals in therapy while the therapist assesses interactions and provides guidance and opportunity for parental success in refeeding the patient. The adolescent's autonomy in other life areas, such as school and social domains, are kept intact, with appropriate supervision consistent with the patient's stage of development.

In the second phase of treatment, control over eating is shifted to the adolescent. Criteria for determining this shift include the patient's weight, which needs to be at least 87% of ideal. The adolescent also needs to show evidence of eating without undue prompting or a struggle with parents. Parents should feel empowered through the refeeding process, and the patient should feel relief that he or she can manage it from here forward.

Once eating and weight disturbances, and other symptomatic behavior, are convincingly under control, then phase three begins. In this phase, the family is prepared for termination of therapy. Issues of importance to the patient are addressed. The family is taught how to use problem solving to address difficulties. Planning for possible future issues is reviewed, and the family is taught how to use skills learned in the therapy to address issues if they arise.

The three phases of FBT for AN are summarized in Figure 4.1.

As Division 12 notes, FBT views the parents of adolescents with AN as a resource for resolving the problem. It corrects misappraisals of blame directed to the parents and to the ill adolescent. Siblings are guided to play a supportive role in treatment, but they are assigned no job role in the refeeding process. The focus of FBT is not on the presumed causes of AN, but rather on how the family can use its strengths to reverse unhealthy beliefs and practices while developing and maintaining new healthy ones around eating, weight, and health. Although FBT has shown efficacy in the short- and long-term treatment of AN, reviewers have commented that its mechanisms of action remain unclear. The call for further study of these mechanisms has been sounded.

Cognitive–Behavioral Therapy (CBT) for Anorexia Nervosa

While FBT has emerged as an evidence-based treatment for adolescents with AN, there is a clear need to develop effective treatments for older adolescents and adults with the disorder. Outcome studies to date have yielded only modest results and often have high dropout rates and other methodological issues that limit conclusions. To date, while most reviewers of this literature acknowledge the need for further study, some, such as APA's Division 12, have noted that cognitive-behavioral therapy has received preliminary support for treating AN when it is used in a particular manner. They currently judge it as probably efficacious.

Figure 4.1

The Three Phases of Family-Based Treatment for Anorexia Nervosa

PHASE 1:

- Parents are placed in charge of the nutritional rehabilitation and weight restoration of the adolescent.
- "The family meal" serves as an arena for assessment and intervention.
- The adolescent's autonomy in other life areas, such as school and social domains, are kept intact.

PHASE 2:

- Control over eating is shifted to the adolescent.
- Progress to this phase is based on sufficient patient weight gain.
- There should be evidence of eating without undue prompting or a struggle with parents.
- Parents should feel empowered.
- The patient should feel relief that he or she can manage the feeding process.

PHASE 3:

- Family is prepared for termination of therapy.
- Important adolescent issues are reviewed.
- Use of problem solving is taught.
- Possible future issues are planned for.
- Use of therapy skills to address issues is reviewed.

Figure 4.2

ESTs for Anorexia Nervosa (AN)

- Well-Established:
  - Family-based treatment

- Probably Efficacious:
  - Cognitive-behavioral therapy

Figure 4.3

Features of Cognitive–Behavioral Therapy for Anorexia Nervosa

- Establishing a regular pattern of eating
- Systematic exposure to "forbidden foods"
- Addressing motivational factors
- Using cognitive restructuring of distorted beliefs about body shape and weight, as well as the tie between personal identity and AN

CBT for AN is intended for late adolescents and adults as a post-hospitalization outpatient intervention designed to prevent relapse once the patient has gained sufficient weight in the context of inpatient treatment. This specification for its use is partly based on the mixed results it has shown as an intervention for restoring weight. CBT for AN is typically conducted as an individual therapy over the course of one year. The therapy begins with biweekly sessions and moves to a weekly schedule once healthy weight is restored and stabilized. Behavioral strategies used in this therapy include establishing a regular pattern of eating as well as exposure to what the patient has seen as "forbidden foods." It also addresses motivational factors and cognitive biases related to the patient's appraisal of shape and weight. Cognitive interventions typically target change in deeper belief systems that support the strong tie between the patient's personal identity and the AN.

The features of CBT for AN are summarized in Figure 4.3.

ESTs for Bulimia Nervosa

In contrast to the comparatively underdeveloped evidence base for the treatment of AN, several well-designed treatment outcome studies constitute the evidence base for the treatment of bulimia nervosa (BN). Reviewers of this literature have been highly uniform in the conclusions they have drawn regarding evidence-based psychological treatments. For example, APA's Division 12 has identified two treatments as well-established and one as probably efficacious for the treatment of BN. The two well-established treatments are cognitive-behavioral therapy (CBT) and interpersonal therapy (IPT). Family-based treatment, adapted from the Maudsley Model we have just discussed for AN, has also shown promise in treating BN. It is currently judged by Division 12 as probably efficacious. Other reviewers, such as the AHRQ, the NICE in Great Britain, the Cochrane Reviews, and Wilson and Fairburn (2007) in Nathan and Gorman's series, *A Guide to Treatments that Work,* have drawn similar conclusions regarding these treatments, but point out that the effects of IPT may take longer to emerge relative to CBT.

Figure 4.4 lists the ESTs for the treatment of BN.

Figure 4.4

ESTs for Bulimia Nervosa

- Well-Established:
  - Cognitive-behavioral therapy
  - Interpersonal therapy

- Probably Efficacious:
  - Family-based treatment

Cognitive–Behavioral Therapy for Bulimia Nervosa

Cognitive-behavioral therapy (CBT) for BN directly targets the core features of this disorder, namely the binge eating, the unhealthy compensatory behaviors such as purging, and the excessive concern with body shape and weight. The treatment focuses on how these features operate in the present to maintain the disorder, as opposed to why they originally developed.

CBT for BN is administered in three phases. The first phase involves psychoeducation regarding weight and the adverse physiological effects of binge eating, purging, extreme dieting, and the like. It encourages the patient to establish a regular pattern of eating and an appropriate weight-monitoring schedule, such as weekly instead of multiple times daily. Stimulus control procedures, such as eliminating binge foods from the house, confining eating to specific times and places, and not shopping for food when especially hungry, are typically employed. Self-control strategies, such as replacing binging with alternative, pleasurable, and feasible activities like talking with a friend, taking a walk, and listening to music, are explained and implemented.

In the second phase of treatment, the focus shifts to eliminating dieting, reducing shape and weight concerns through cognitive restructuring, and learning problem solving to manage stresses as opposed to using binging.

The third phase is devoted to developing a maintenance plan and to the prevention of relapse using common considerations.

The three phases of CBT for BN are summarized in Figure 4.5.

Interpersonal Therapy for Bulimia Nervosa

Interpersonal therapy (IPT) for BN is based on the treatment that was originally developed and subsequently shown to be efficacious for the treatment of depression. In IPT, the focus of therapy is on resolving interpersonal difficulties in the patient's life as opposed to directly treating the eating disorder explicitly. The relationship between interpersonal problems and the eating disorder is identified during the initial phase of treatment, but it's only implied thereafter.

Figure 4.5

The Three Phases of Cognitive–Behavioral Therapy for Bulimia Nervosa

PHASE 1

- Psychoeducation on the adverse effects of binging, purging, and extreme dieting
- Encourages a regular pattern of eating and reasonable weight-monitoring frequency
- Stimulus control procedures applied to eating times and places, food shopping times
- Self-control strategies address healthy alternative activities to binging

PHASE 2

- Cognitive restructuring targeting dieting, shape and weight concerns
- Problem solving to manage causes of stress

PHASE 3

- Development of a maintenance plan
- Implements relapse prevention strategies

The first phase is devoted to thoroughly assessing the eating disorder as well as significant past and present interpersonal relationships. This assessment is called the Interpersonal Inventory. The therapist leads this question-and-answer, back-and-forth assessment. Although interpersonal precipitants of current binge-eating episodes are identified, the interpersonal issues are targeted for later treatment. A specific interpersonal problem or problems are agreed upon in Phase 1, and they become the focus of the second phase of treatment.

Common themes of the second phase of IPT include role disputes, role transitions, interpersonal deficits, and unresolved grief. In this second phase of treatment, the role of the therapist and client shift, as the client takes the lead by discussing and being willing to explore change in the interpersonal problems identified in Phase 1. IPT therapists lean on techniques traditionally associated with nondirective client-centered therapies to help clarify issues being raised by the patient. They also keep the patient focused on the problem and encourage the client's willingness to change. They may also use techniques that are traditionally associated with behavioral therapies, such as role-plays and problem solving, when dealing with how a particular change in interpersonal functioning might be accomplished by the client.

The third phase of this treatment typically emphasizes maintaining therapeutic gains and preventing relapse.

Figure 4.6 summarizes the three phases of IPT for BN.

Figure 4.6

The Three Phases of Interpersonal Therapy for Bulimia Nervosa

PHASE 1: THERAPIST LEADS

- Assessment of bulimia
- Taking Interpersonal Inventory of past and present relationships
- Agreeing on a problem or problems to focus on during Phase 2

PHASE 2: CLIENT LEADS

- Themes: role disputes, role transitions, interpersonal deficits, unresolved grief
- Client explores clarification and change in interpersonal problems
- Nondirective techniques are used to facilitate the process
- Role-play and problem solving may be used

PHASE 3

- Consolidation of gains
- Relapse prevention

ESTs for Binge-Eating Disorder

As with BN, several reviewers have identified CBT and IPT as evidence-based treatments for binge-eating disorder (BED). For example, APA's Division 12 notes that these two treatments are the only two that have an evidence base sufficient to meet their criteria for a well-established treatment. Other reviewers (e.g., Wilson & Fairburn, 2007), using criteria involving high-quality trials but not requiring independent replication as does Division 12, have noted that these and other treatments such as behavioral weight loss programs and guided self-help using CBT principles have shown efficacy for BED treatment. However, these reviewers note that the efficacy for treatments other than CBT and IPT has been demonstrated in short-term trials only. CBT and IPT are the only treatments that have demonstrated replicated efficacy for BED in both short- and longer-term trials. Figure 4.7 lists the ESTs for BED treatment.

Figure 4.7

ESTs for Binge-Eating Disorder

- Cognitive-behavioral therapy
- Interpersonal therapy

Obesity

Many professional medical organizations have developed evidence-based practice guidelines for assessing and treating obesity, including family medicine and pediatrics. These guidelines emphasize the importance of multicomponent interventions focused on changes in lifestyle, diet, and exercise. The guidelines from NICE in Great Britain similarly conclude that these multicomponent interventions are the treatment of choice for overweight and obesity. They recommend that weight management programs include behavior change strategies to increase people's physical activity levels, as well as improve their eating behavior and the quality of their diet. Examples of recommended behavior change strategies are those well-known to behavioral medicine and include self-monitoring of behavior and progress, stimulus control procedures (such as setting regular meal times and removing access to high-calorie "junk foods"), as well as more traditional cognitive-behavioral objectives such as learning how to problem solve, learning and implementing communication/assertiveness skills, practicing cognitive restructuring, ensuring social support, and learning and implementing relapse prevention strategies.

EST for Obesity Treatment

Division 12 of the APA has identified Behavioral Weight Loss (BWL) treatments for obesity as the only type of intervention for obesity that has met its criteria for a well-established treatment. They note that BWL is a short-term treatment that uses many of the interventions noted previously to achieve acute weight reduction and establish new behavioral patterns aimed at maintaining the weight loss. They cite the LEARN model as an exemplar of this approach.

Behavioral Weight Loss (LEARN Model)

LEARN is an acronym that reflects the multicomponent emphasis of this well-studied version of BWL. It stands for Lifestyle, Exercise, Attitudes, Relationships, and Nutrition. The program promotes changes in these multiple domains designed to synergistically yield and maintain weight loss. LEARN can be conceptualized, and is often delivered, as a series of lessons that break down its five major themes. Among its emphases, it (1) encourages setting reasonable expectations and weight goals; (2) teaches healthy nutrition; (3) prescribes variety in food choices (no food is completely forbidden, but rather moderation in consumption is emphasized); (4) encourages small changes in daily lifestyle activity; and (5) teaches cognitive restructuring and behavioral skills such as communication, problem solving, and relapse prevention.

Figure 4.8 lists primary emphases of LEARN program for obesity treatment

Figure 4.8

Emphases of LEARN for Obesity Treatment

- Sets reasonable expectations and weight goals
- Teaches healthy nutrition
- Prescribes variety and moderation in food choices
- Encourages small changes in daily lifestyle activity
- Teaches cognitive restructuring
- Teaches behavioral skills such as communication, problem solving, and relapse prevention

Chapter Review

1. As presented in this chapter, what are the empirically supported psychological treatments for Anorexia Nervosa?
2. What are the three phases of family-based treatment for anorexia nervosa?
3. What are the features of cognitive behavioral therapy for anorexia nervosa?
4. What are the empirically supported psychological treatments for bulimia nervosa?
5. What are the three phases of cognitive-behavioral therapy for bulimia nervosa?
6. What are the three phases of interpersonal therapy for bulimia?
7. What are the empirically supported psychological treatments for binge-eating disorder?
8. What are key emphases of the behavioral weight loss program LEARN?

Chapter Review Test Questions

1. According to APA's Division 12, The Society of Clinical Psychology, which of the following has met their criteria for a well-established psychological treatment for anorexia nervosa (AN)?

   A. Cognitive-behavioral therapy (CBT)
   B. Interpersonal therapy (IPT)
   C. Family-based treatment (FBT)
   D. Supportive psychotherapy (SP)

2. Which of the following is *not* one of the empirically supported treatments for bulimia nervosa (BN) cited by APA's Division 12, The Society of Clinical Psychology?

   A. Cognitive-behavioral therapy (CBT)
   B. Interpersonal therapy (IPT)
   C. Family-based treatment (FBT)
   D. Supportive psychotherapy (SP)

Selected Chapter References

General and Reviews

Hay, P. J. (2008). Eating disorders. In J. A. Trafton & W. Gordon (Eds.), *Best practices in the behavioral management of health from preconception to adolescence*. Los Altos, CA: The Institute for Brain Potential.

Hudson, J. I., Hiripi, E., Pope, H. G., & Kessler, R. C. (2007). The prevalence and correlates of eating disorders in the national comorbidity survey replication. *Biological Psychiatry, 61*, 348–358.

Keel, P. K., & Haedt, A. (2008). Evidence-based psychosocial treatments for eating problems and eating disorders. *Journal of Clinical Child & Adolescent Psychology, 37*, 39–61.

Wilson, G. T., & Fairburn, C. G. (2007). Treatments for eating disorders. In P. E. Nathan & J. M. Gorman (Eds.), *A guide to treatments that work* (3rd ed., pp. 579–610). New York, NY: Oxford University Press.

Wilson, G. T., Grilo, C. M., & Vitousek, K. M. (2007). Psychological treatment of eating disorders. *American Psychologist, 62*(3), 199–216.

Anorexia Nervosa

Family-Based Therapy

Empirical Support

Eisler, I., Dare, C., Hodes, M., Russell, G. F. M., Dodge, E., & le Grange, D. (2000). Family therapy for adolescent anorexia nervosa: The results of a controlled comparison of two family interventions. *Journal of Child Psychology and Psychiatry, 41*, 727–736.

Eisler, I., Dare, C., Russell, G. F. M., Szmukler, G. I., le Grange, D., & Dodge, E. (1997). Family and individual therapy in anorexia nervosa: A five-year follow-up. *Archives of General Psychiatry, 54*, 1025–1030.

Eisler, I., Simic, M., Russell, G. F. M., & Dare, C. (2007). A randomized controlled treatment trial of two forms of family therapy in adolescent anorexia nervosa: A five year follow-up. *Journal of Child Psychology and Psychiatry, 48*(6), 552–560.

Le Grange, D., Binford, R., & Loeb, K. L. (2005). Manualized family-based treatment for adolescent anorexia nervosa: A case series. *Journal of the American Academy of Child and Adolescent Psychiatry, 44*, 41–46.

Le Grange, D., Eisler, I., Dare, C., & Russell, G. F. M. (1992). Evaluation of family treatments in adolescent anorexia nervosa: A pilot study. *International Journal of Eating Disorders, 12*, 347–357.

Lock, J., le Grange, D., Forsberg, S., & Hewell, K. (2006). Is family therapy useful for treating children with anorexia nervosa? Results of a case series. *Journal of the American Academy of Child and Adolescent Psychiatry, 45*(11), 1323–1328.

Lock, J., Couturier, J., & Agras, W. S. (2006). Comparison of long term outcomes in adolescents with anorexia nervosa treated with family therapy. *Academy of Child and Adolescent Psychiatry, 45,* 666–672.

Lock, J., Agras, W. S., Bryson, S., & Kraemer, H. C. (2005). A comparison of short- and long-term family therapy for adolescent anorexia nervosa. *Academy of Child and Adolescent Psychiatry, 44,* 632–639.

Lock, J., le Grange, D., Agras, W. S., Moye, A., Bryson, S. W., & Jo, B. (2010). Randomized clinical trial comparing family-based treatment with adolescent-focused individual therapy for adolescents with anorexia nervosa. *Archives of General Psychiatry, 67*(10), 1025–1032.

Loeb, K. L., Walsh, T. B., Lock, J., le Grange, D., Jones, J., Marcus, S., . . . Dobrow, I. (2007). Open trial of family-based treatment for full and partial anorexia nervosa in adolescence: Evidence of successful dissemination. *Journal of the American Academy of Child and Adolescent Psychiatry, 46*(7), 792–800.

Robin, A. L., Siegel, P. T., Moye, A. W., Gilroy, M., Dennis, A. B., & Sikand, A. (1999). A controlled comparison of family versus individual therapy for adolescents with anorexia nervosa. *Journal of the American Academy of Child and Adolescent Psychiatry, 38*(12), 1482–1489.

Robin, A. L., Siegel, P. T., Koepke, T., Moye, A. W., & Tice, S. (1994). Family therapy versus individual therapy for adolescent females with anorexia nervosa. *Journal of Developmental and Behavioral Pediatrics, 15*(2), 111–116.

Russell, G. F. M., Szmukler, G. I., Dare, C., & Eisler, I. (1987). An evaluation of family therapy in anorexia nervosa and bulimia nervosa. *Archives of General Psychiatry 44,* 1047–1056.

Clinical Resources

Lock, J., le Grange, D., Agras, W. S., & Dare, C. (2001). *Treatment manual for anorexia nervosa: A family-based approach.* New York, NY: Guilford Press.

Training Opportunities

Daniel le Grange, Ph.D., The University of Chicago, legrange@uchicago.edu
James Lock, MD, Ph.D., Stanford University, jimlock@stanford.edu
Note: Training opportunities information from www.psycholoicaltreatments.org.
Katharine L. Loeb, Ph.D., Fairleigh Dickinson University and Mount Sinai School of Medicine, katharine.loeb@mssm.edu

Cognitive–Behavioral Therapy

Empirical Support

Halmi, K. A., Agras, W. S., Crow, S., Mitchell, J., Wilson, G. T., Bryson, S. W., & Kraemer, H. C. (2005). Predictors of treatment acceptance and completion in anorexia nervosa: Implications for future study designs. *Archives of General Psychiatry, 62*(7), 776–781.

McIntosh, V. V. W., Jordan, J., Carter, F., Luty, S. E., McKenzie, J. M., Bulik, C. M., . . . Joyce, P. R. (2005). Three psychotherapies for anorexia nervosa: A randomized, controlled trial. *American Journal of Psychiatry 162*, 741–747.

Pike, K. M., Walsh, B. T., Vitousek, K., Wilson, G. T., & Bauer, J. (2003). Cognitive behavior therapy in the posthospitalization treatment of anorexia nervosa. *American Journal of Psychiatry, 160*, 2046–2049.

Walsh, B. T., Kaplan, A. S., Attia, E., Olmstead, M., Parides, M., Carter, J. C., . . . Rockert, W. (2006). Fluoxetine after weight restoration in anorexia nervosa: A randomized controlled trial. *Journal of the American Medical Association, 295*, 2605–2612.

Clinical Resources

Garner, D. M., Vitousek, K. M., & Pike, K. M. (1997). Cognitive-behavioral therapy for anorexia nervosa. In D. M. Garner & P. E. Garfinkel (Eds.), *Handbook of treatment for eating disorders* (2nd ed., pp. 94–144). New York, NY: The Guilford Press.

Pike, K. M., Devlin, M. J., & Loeb, K. L. (2004). Cognitive-behavioral therapy in the treatment of anorexia nervosa, bulimia nervosa, and binge eating disorder. In J. K. Thompson (Ed.), *Handbook of eating disorders and obesity* (pp. 130–162). Hoboken, NJ: Wiley.

Training Opportunities

Christopher G. Fairburn, DM, FRCPsych, Oxford University, credo@medsci.ox.ac.uk
Kathleen M. Pike, PhD, Columbia University, kmp2@columbia.edu

Bulimia Nervosa

Cognitive-Behavioral Therapy

Empirical Support

Agras, W., Rossiter, E., Arnow, B., Schneider, J., Telch, C., Raeburn, S., . . . Koran, L. M. (1992). Pharmacologic and cognitive-behavioral treatment for bulimia nervosa: A controlled comparison. *American Journal of Psychiatry, 149*, 82–87.

Agras, W. S., Rossiter, E. M., Arnow, B., Telch, C. F., Raeburn, S. D., Bruce, B., & Koran, L. (1994). One-year follow up of psychosocial and pharmacologic treatments for bulimia nervosa. *Journal of Clinical Psychiatry, 55*, 179–183.

Agras, W. S., Schneider, J. A., Arnow, B., Raeburn, S. D., & Telch, C. F. (1989). Cognitive-behavioral and response-prevention treatments for bulimia nervosa. *Journal of Consulting and Clinical Psychology, 57*, 215–221.

Agras, W. S., Walsh, T., Fairburn, C. G., Wilson, G. T., & Kraemer, H. C. (2000). A multicenter comparison of cognitive-behavioral therapy and interpersonal psychotherapy for bulimia nervosa. *Archives of General Psychiatry, 57*(5), 459–466.

Bailer, U., deZwaan, M., Leisch, F., Strnad, A., Lennkh-Wolfsberg, C., El-Giamal, N., . . . Kasper, S. (2004). Guided self-help versus cognitive-behavioral group therapy in the treatment of bulimia nervosa. *International Journal of Eating Disorders, 35*, 522–537.

Banasiak, S. J., Paxton, S. J., & Hay, P. (2005). Guided self-help for bulimia nervosa in primary care: A randomized controlled trial. *Psychological Medicine, 35*(9), 1283–1294.

Bulik, C., Sullivan, P., Carter, F., McIntosh, V., & Joyce, P. (1998). The role of exposure with response prevention in the cognitive-behavioral therapy for bulimia nervosa. *Psychological Medicine, 28*, 611–623.

Carter, F., McIntosh, V., Joyce, P., Sullivan, P., & Bulik, C. (2003). Role of exposure with response prevention in cognitive-behavioral therapy for bulimia nervosa: Three-year follow-up results. *International Journal of Eating Disorders, 33*, 127–135.

Carter, J., Olmstead, M., Kaplan, A., McCabe, R., Mills, J., & Aime, A. (2003). Self-help for bulimia nervosa: A randomized controlled trial. *American Journal of Psychiatry, 160*, 973–978.

Chen, E., Touyz, S., Beumont, P., Fairburn, C., Griffiths, R., Butow, P., . . . Basten, C. (2003). Comparison of group and individual cognitive-behavioral therapy for bulimia nervosa. *International Journal of Eating Disorders, 33*, 241–254.

Cooper, P., & Steere, J. (1995). A comparison of two psychological treatments for bulimia nervosa: Implications for models of maintenance. *Behaviour Research and Therapy, 33*, 875–885.

Durand, M., & King, M. (2003). Specialist treatment versus self-help for bulimia nervosa: A randomised control trial in general practice. *British Journal of General Practice, 53*, 371–377.

Fairburn, C. G., Cooper, Z., & Shafran, R. (2003). Cognitive behaviour therapy for eating disorders: A "transdiagnostic" theory and treatment. *Behaviour Research and Therapy, 41*(5), 509–528.

Fairburn, C. G., Jones, R., Peveler, R. C., Carr, S. J., Solomon, R. A., O'Connor, M. E., . . . Hope, R. A. (1991). Three psychological treatments for bulimia nervosa: A comparative trial. *Archives of General Psychiatry, 48*, 463–469.

Fairburn, C. G., Jones, R., Peveler, R. C., Hope, R. A., & O'Connor, M. (1993). Psychotherapy and bulimia nervosa: The longer-term effects of interpersonal psychotherapy, behaviour therapy and cognitive behaviour therapy. *Archives of General Psychiatry, 50*, 419–428.

Fairburn, C. G., Kirk, J., O'Connor, M., & Cooper, P. J. (1986). A comparison of two psychological treatments for bulimia nervosa. *Behaviour Research and Therapy, 24,* 629–643.

Fairburn, C. G., Norman, P. A., Welch, S. L., O'Connor, M. E., Doll, H. A., & Peveler, R. C. (1995). A prospective study of outcome in bulimia nervosa and the long-term effects of three psychological treatments. *Archives of General Psychiatry, 52,* 304–312.

Garner, D., Rockert, W., Davis, R., Garner, M., Olmstead, M., & Eagle, M. (1993). Comparison of cognitive-behavioral and supportive-expressive therapy for bulimia nervosa. *American Journal of Psychiatry, 150,* 37–46.

Goldbloom, D. S., Olmstead, M., Davis, R., Clewes, J., Heinmaa, M., Rockert, W., & Shaw, B. (1997). A randomized controlled trial of fluoxetine and cognitive behavioral therapy for bulimia nervosa: Short-term outcome. *Behaviour Research and Therapy, 35,* 803–811.

Hsu, L. K., Rand, W., Sullivan, S., Liu, D.W., Mulliken, B., McDonagh, B., & Kaye, W. H. (2001). Cognitive therapy, nutritional therapy and their combination in the treatment of bulimia nervosa. *Psychological Medicine, 31,* 871–879.

Lock, J. (2005). Adjusting cognitive behavior therapy for adolescents with bulimia nervosa: Results of case series. *American Journal of Psychotherapy, 59*(3), 267–281.

Mitchell, J. E., Fletcher, L., Hanson, K., Mussell, M. P., Seim, H., Crosby, R., & Al-Banna, M. (2001). The relative efficacy of fluoxetine and manual-based self-help in the treatment of outpatients with bulimia nervosa. *Journal of Clinical Psychopharmacology, 21,* 298–304.

Mitchell, J. E., Halmi, K., Wilson, G. T., Agras, W. S., Kraemer, H., & Crow, S. (2002). A randomized secondary treatment study of women with bulimia nervosa who fail to respond to CBT. *International Journal of Eating Disorders, 32*(3), 271–281.

Nevonen, L., & Broberg, A. G. (2006). A comparison of sequenced individual and group psychotherapy for patients with bulimia nervosa. *International Journal of Eating Disorders, 39*(2), 117–127.

Schapman-Williams, A. M., Lock, J., & Couturier, J. (2006). Cognitive-behavioral therapy for adolescents with binge eating syndromes: A case series. *International Journal of Eating Disorders, 39*(3), 252–255.

Schmidt, U., Lee, S., Beecham, J., Perkins, S., Treasure, J., Yi, I., . . . Eisler, I. (2007). A randomized controlled trial of family therapy and cognitive behavior therapy guided self-care for adolescents with bulimia nervosa and related disorders. *American Journal of Psychiatry, 164,* 591–598.

Sungot-Borgen, J., Rosenvinge, J. H., Bahr, R., & Schneider, L. S. (2002). The effect of exercise, cognitive therapy, and nutritional counseling in treating bulimia nervosa. *Medicine and Science in Sports and Exercise, 34,* 190–195.

Thiels, C., Schmidt, U., Treasure, J., Garthe, R., & Troop, N. (1998). Guided self-change for bulimia nervosa incorporating the use of a self-care manual. *American Journal of Psychiatry, 155,* 947–953.

Walsh, B. T., Fairburn, C. G., Mickley, D., Sysko, R., & Parides, M. K. (2004). Treatment of bulimia nervosa in a primary care setting. *American Journal of Psychiatry, 161,* 556–561.

Walsh, B. T., Wilson, G. T., Loeb, K. L., Devlin, M. J., Pike, K. M., Roose, S. P., . . . Waternaux, C. (1997). Medication and psychotherapy in the treatment of bulimia nervosa. *American Journal of Psychiatry, 154,* 523–531.

Clinical Resources

Fairburn, C. G. (2008). *Cognitive behavior therapy and eating disorders.* New York, NY: Guilford Press.

Fairburn, C. G. (1995). *Overcoming binge eating.* New York, NY: Guilford Press.

Fairburn, C. G., Marcus, M. D., & Wilson, G. T. (1993). Cognitive-behavioral therapy for binge eating and bulimia nervosa: A comprehensive treatment manual. In C. G. Fairburn & G. T. Wilson (Eds.), *Binge eating: Nature, assessment and treatment* (pp. 361–404). New York, NY: Guilford Press.

Training Opportunities

Christopher G. Fairburn, DM, FRCPsych, Oxford University, credo@medsci.ox.ac.uk

Interpersonal Therapy

Empirical Support

Agras, W. S., Walsh, T., Fairburn, C. G., Wilson, G. T., & Kraemer, H. C. (2000). A multicenter comparison of cognitive-behavioral therapy and interpersonal psychotherapy for bulimia nervosa. *Archives of General Psychiatry, 57*(5), 459–466.

Fairburn, C. G., Norman, P. A., Welch, S. L., O'Connor, M. E., Doll, H. A., & Peveler, R. C. (1995). A prospective study of outcome in bulimia nervosa and the long-term effects of three psychological treatments. *Archives of General Psychiatry, 52,* 304–312.

Fairburn, C. G., Jones, R., Peveler, R. C., Hope, R. A., & O'Connor, M. (1993). Psychotherapy and bulimia nervosa: The longer-term effects of interpersonal psychotherapy, behaviour therapy and cognitive behaviour therapy. *Archives of General Psychiatry, 50,* 419–428.

Fairburn, C. G., Jones, R., Peveler, R. C., Carr, S. J., Solomon, R. A., O'Connor, M. E., . . . Hope, R. A. (1991). Three psychological treatments for bulimia nervosa: A comparative trial. *Archives of General Psychiatry, 48,* 463–469.

Fairburn, C. G., Kirk, J., O'Connor, M., & Cooper, P. J. (1986). A comparison of two psychological treatments for bulimia nervosa. *Behaviour Research and Therapy, 24*, 629–643.

Mitchell, J. E., Halmi, K., Wilson, G. T., Agras, W. S., Kraemer, H., & Crow, S. (2002). A randomized secondary treatment study of women with bulimia nervosa who fail to respond to CBT. *International Journal of Eating Disorders, 32*(3), 271–281.

Nevonen, L., & Broberg, A. G. (2006). A comparison of sequenced individual and group psychotherapy for patients with bulimia nervosa. *International Journal of Eating Disorders, 39*(2), 117–127.

Clinical Resources

Fairburn, C. G. (1992). Interpersonal psychotherapy for bulimia nervosa. In G. L. Klerman & M. W. Weissman (Eds.), *New applications of interpersonal psychotherapy* (pp. 353–378). Washington, DC: American Psychiatric Press.

Fairburn, C. G. (1997). Interpersonal psychotherapy for bulimia nervosa. In D. M. Garner & P. E. Garfinkel (Eds.), *Handbook of treatment for eating disorders* (2nd ed., pp. 278–294). New York, NY: The Guilford Press.

Klerman, G. L., Weissman, M. M., Rounsaville, B. J., & Chevron, E. S. (1984). *Interpersonal psychotherapy of depression.* New York, NY: Basic Books.

Training Opportunities

Christopher G. Fairburn, DM, FRCPsych (Oxford University), credo@medsci.ox.ac.uk

Family-Based Treatment

Empirical Support

Le Grange, D., Crosby, R. D., Rathouz, P. J., & Leventhal, B. L. (2007). A randomized controlled comparison of family-based treatment and supportive psychotherapy for adolescent bulimia nervosa. *Archives of General Psychiatry, 64*, 1049–1056.

Schmidt, U., Lee, S., Beecham, J., Perkins, S., Treasure, J., Yi, I., . . . Eisler, I. (2007). A randomized controlled trial of family therapy and cognitive behavior therapy guided self-care for adolescents with bulimia nervosa and related disorders. *American Journal of Psychiatry, 164*, 591–598.

Clinical Resources

Le Grange, D., & Lock, J. (2007). *Treating bulimia in adolescents: A family-based approach.* New York, NY: Guilford Press.

Le Grange, D., & Lock, J. (2011). *Eating disorders in children and adolescents: A clinical handbook.* New York, NY: Guilford Press.

Training Opportunities

Daniel le Grange, PhD, The University of Chicago, legrange@uchicago.edu

James Lock, MD, PhD, Stanford University, jimlock@stanford.edu

Binge–Eating Disorder

Cognitive–Behavioral Therapy

Empirical Support

Agras, W. S., Telch, C. F., Arnow, B., Eldridge, K., Wifley, D. E., Raeburn, S. D., . . . Marnell, M. (1994). Weight loss, cognitive-behavioral, and desipramine treatments in binge eating disorder: An additive design. *Behavior Therapy, 25*, 225–238.

Devlin, M. J., Goldfein, J. A., Petkova, E., Jiang, H., Raizman, P. S., . . . Walsh, T. (2005). Cognitive behavioral therapy and fluoxetine as adjuncts to group behavioral therapy for binge eating disorder. *Obesity Research, 13*(6), 1077–1088.

Gorin, A., le Grange, D., & Stone, A. (2003). Effectiveness of spouse involvement in cognitive behavioral therapy for binge eating disorder. *International Journal of Eating Disorders, 33*, 421–433.

Grilo, C. M., & Masheb, R. M. (2005). A randomized controlled comparison of guided self-help cognitive behavioral therapy and behavioral weight loss for binge eating disorder. *Behaviour Research and Therapy, 43*(11), 1509–1525.

Grilo, C. M., Masheb, R. M., & Salant, S. L. (2005). Cognitive behavioral therapy guided self-help and orlistat for the treatment of binge eating disorder: A randomized, double-blind, placebo-controlled trial. *Biological Psychiatry, 57*, 1193–1201.

Grilo, C. M., Masheb, R. M., & Wilson, G. T. (2005). Efficacy of cognitive behavioral therapy and fluoxetine for the treatment of binge eating disorder: A randomized double-blind placebo-controlled comparison. *Biological Psychiatry, 57*, 301–309.

Hilbert, A., & Tuschen-Caffier, B. (2004). Body image interventions in cognitive-behaviourial therapy of binge eating disorder: A component analysis. *Behaviour Research and Therapy, 42*, 1325–1339.

Munsch, S., Biedert, E., Meyer, A., Michael, T., Schlup, B., Tuch, A., & Margraf, J. (2007). A randomized comparison of cognitive behavioral therapy and behavioral weight loss treatment for overweight individuals with binge eating disorder. *International Journal of Eating Disorders, 40*(2), 102–113.

Telch, C. F., Agras, W. S., Rossiter, E. M., Wilfley, D., & Kenardy, J. (1990). Group cognitive-behavioral treatment for the nonpurging bulimic: An initial evaluation. *Journal of Consulting and Clinical Psychology, 58*(5), 629–635.

Wilfley, D. E., Agras, W. S., Telch, C. F., Rossiter, E. M., Schneider, J. A., Cole, A. G., . . . Raeburn, S. D. (1993). Group cognitive-behavioral therapy and group interpersonal psychotherapy for the nonpurging bulimic individual: A controlled comparison. *Journal of Consulting and Clinical Psychology, 61*, 296–305.

Wilfley, D. E., Welch, R. R., Stein, R. I., Spurrell, E. B., Cohen, L. R., Saelens, B. E., . . . Matt, G. E. (2002). A randomized comparison of group cognitive-behavioral therapy and group interpersonal psychotherapy for the treatment of overweight individuals with binge-eating disorder. *Archives of General Psychiatry, 59*(8), 713–721.

Clinical Resources

Grilo, C. M., & Mitchell, J. E. (2011). *The treatment of eating disorders: A clinical handbook*. New York, NY: Guilford Press.

Fairburn, C. G. (1995). *Overcoming binge eating*. New York, NY: Guilford Press.

Fairburn, C. G., Marcus, M. D., & Wilson, G. T. (1993). Cognitive-behavioral therapy for binge eating and bulimia nervosa: A comprehensive treatment manual. In C. G. Fairburn & G. T. Wilson (Eds.), *Binge eating: Nature, assessment and treatment* (pp. 361–404). New York, NY: Guilford Press.

Marcus, M. (1997). Adapting treatment for patients with binge eating disorder. In D. M. Garner & P. E. Garfinkel (Eds.), *Handbook of treatment for eating disorders* (2nd ed., pp. 484–493). New York, NY: Guilford Press.

Wilfley, D. E., Grilo, C. M., & Rodin, J. (1997). Group psychotherapy for the treatment of bulimia nervosa and binge eating disorder: Research and clinical methods. In J. L. Spira (Ed.), *Group therapy for medically ill patients* (pp. 225–295). New York, NY: Guilford Press.

Training Opportunities

Michael J. Devlin, M.D., Columbia University, mjd5@columbia.edu

Christopher G. Fairburn, D.M., FRCPsych, Oxford University, credo@medsci.ox.ac.uk

Carlos Grilo, Ph.D., Yale University, carlos.grilo@yale.edu

Interpersonal Therapy

Empirical Support

Wilfley, D. E., Agras, W. S., Telch, C. F., Rossiter, E. M., Schneider, J. A., Cole, A. G., . . . Raeburn, S. D. (1993). Group cognitive-behavioral therapy and group interpersonal psychotherapy for the nonpurging bulimic individual: A controlled comparison. *Journal of Consulting and Clinical Psychology, 61*, 296–305.

Wilfley, D. E., Welch, R. R., Stein, R. I., Spurrell, E. B., Cohen, L. R., Saelens, B. E., . . . Matt, G. E. (2002). A randomized comparison of group cognitive-behavioral therapy and group interpersonal psychotherapy for the treatment of overweight individuals with binge-eating disorder. *Archives of General Psychiatry, 59*(8), 713–721.

Wilson, G. T., Wilfley, D. E., Agras, W. S., & Bryson, S. W. (2010).Psychological treatments for binge eating disorder. *Archives of General Psychiatry, 67*, 94–101.

Clinical Resources

Klerman, G. L., Weissman, M. M., Rounsaville, B. J., & Chevron, E. S. (1984). *Interpersonal psychotherapy of depression*. New York, NY: Basic Books.

Wilfley, D. E., Grilo, C. M., & Rodin, J. (1997). Group psychotherapy for the treatment of bulimia nervosa and binge eating disorder: Research and clinical methods. In J. L. Spira (Ed.), *Group therapy for medically ill patients* (pp. 225–295). New York, NY: Guilford Press.

Wilfley, D. E., Mackenzie, K. R., Welch, R., Ayres, V., & Weissman, M. M. (2000). *Interpersonal Psychotherapy for Group*. New York, NY: Basic Books.

Training Opportunities

Christopher G. Fairburn, D.M., FRCPsych, Oxford University, credo@medsci.ox.ac.uk

Obesity

Behavioral Weight Loss (e.g., LEARN)

Empirical Support

Berkowitz, R. I., Wadden, T. A., Tershakovec, A. M., & Cronquist, J. L. (2003) Behavior therapy and sibutramine for treatment of adolescent obesity. *Journal of the American Medical Association, 289*, 1805–1812.

Diabetes Prevention Program Research Group. (2002). Reduction in the incidence of Type 2 diabetes with lifestyle interventions or metformin. *New England Journal of Medicine, 346*, 393–403.

Epstein, L. H., Paluch, R. A., Kilanowski, C. K., & Raynor, H. A. (2004). The effect of reinforcement or stimulus control to reduce sedentary behavior in the treatment of pediatric obesity. *Health Psychology, 23*, 371–380.

Golan, M., Kaufman, V., & Shahar, D. R. (2006). Childhood obesity treatment: Targeting parents exclusively v. parents and children. *British Journal of Nutrition, 95*, 1008–1015.

Hypertension Prevention Trial Research Group. (1990). The hypertension prevention trial: Three-year effects of dietary changes on blood pressure. *Archives of Internal Medicine, 150*, 153–162.

Jeffery, R. W., & Wing, R. R. (1995). Long-term effects of interventions for weight loss using food provision and monetary incentives. *Journal of Consulting and Clinical Psychology, 65,* 793–796.

Wadden, T. A., Foster, G. D., & Letizia, K. A. (1994). One-year behavioral treatment of obesity: Comparison of moderate and severe caloric restriction and the effects of weight maintenance therapy. *Journal of Consulting and Clinical Psychology, 62,* 165–171.

Wadden, T. A., & The Look AHEAD Research Group. (2006). The Look AHEAD study: A description of the lifestyle intervention and the evidence supporting it. *Obesity, 14,* 737–752.

Wadden, T. A., Berkowitz, R. I., Womble, L. G., Sarwer, D. B., Phelan, S., Cato, R. K., . . . Stunkard, A. J. (2005). Randomized trial of lifestyle modification and pharmacotherapy for obesity. *New England Journal of Medicine, 353,* 2111–2120.

Wing, R. R., Blair, E., Marcus, M., Epstein, L. H., & Harvey, J. (1994). Year-long weight loss treatment for obese patients with type II diabetes: Does including an intermittent very-low-calorie diet improve outcome? *American Journal of Medicine, 97,* 354–362.

Clinical Resources

Brownell, K. D. (2004). *The LEARN program for weight management* (10th ed.). Dallas, TX: American Health.

Training Opportunities

The LEARN Institute for Lifestyle Management at http://www.thelifestylecompany.com/lccp/lccp.htm (adults)

Leonard Epstein, Ph.D., State University of New York at Buffalo (children and adolescents) E-mail: lhenet@buffalo.edu

Bibliotherapy Resources

Fairburn, C. G. (1995). *Overcoming binge eating.* New York, NY: Guilford Press.

Lock, J., & le Grange, D. (2005). *Help your teenager beat an eating disorder.* New York, NY: Guilford Press.

Katzman, D. K., & Pinhas, L. (2005). *Help for eating disorders: A parent's guide to symptoms, causes and treatments.* Toronto, Canada: Robert Rose.

Walsh, B. T., & Cameron, V. L. (2005). *If your adolescent has an eating disorder: An essential resource for parents.* New York, NY: Oxford University Press.

Note: Training opportunities information is from www.psychologicaltreatments.org.

5

How Do You Integrate Empirically Supported Treatments Into Treatment Planning?

Construction of an empirically informed treatment plan for Eating Disorders and Obesity involves integrating objectives and treatment interventions consistent with identified empirically supported treatments (ESTs) into a client's treatment plan after you have determined that the client's primary problem fits those described in the target population of the EST research. Of course, implementing ESTs must be done in consideration of important client, therapist, and therapeutic relationship factors—consistent with the APA's definition of evidence-based practice.

Definitions

The behavioral definition statements describe *how the problem manifests itself in the client*. Although there are several common features of eating disorders and obesity, the behavioral definition for your client will be unique and specific to him/her. We begin building our treatment plan for eating disorders and obesity by selecting behavioral definition statements that describe the symptom pattern of our specific client. Examples of behavioral definition statements are the following:

➢ Refusal to maintain body weight at or above a minimally normal weight for age and height (i.e., body weight less than 85% of that expected)
➢ Intense fear of gaining weight or becoming fat, even though underweight
➢ Persistent preoccupation with body image related to grossly inaccurate assessment of self as overweight
➢ Undue influence of body weight or shape on self-evaluation
➢ Strong denial of the seriousness of the current low body weight
➢ In post-menarcheal females, amenorrhea (i.e., the absence of at least three consecutive menstrual cycles)
➢ Escalating fluid and electrolyte imbalance resulting from eating disorder

➤ Recurrent inappropriate compensatory behaviors in order to prevent weight gain, such as self-induced vomiting; misuse of laxatives, diuretics, enemas, or other medications; fasting; or excessive exercise

➤ Recurrent episodes of binge eating (a large amount of food is consumed in a relatively short period, and there is a sense of lack of control over the eating behavior)

➤ Eating much more rapidly than normal

➤ Eating until feeling uncomfortably full

➤ Eating large amounts of food when not feeling physically hungry

➤ Eating alone because of feeling embarrassed by how much one is eating

➤ Feeling disgusted with oneself, depressed, or very guilty after eating too much

➤ An excess of body weight, relative to height, which is attributed to an abnormally high proportion of body fat (Body Mass Index of 30 or more)

The list starts with eight statements that characterize anorexia nervosa. Some of the first statements could also apply to a client struggling with bulimia nervosa, such as "Undue influence of body weight or shape on self-evaluation," but statements such as "Recurrent inappropriate compensatory behaviors and recurrent episodes of binge eating" are most clearly associated with bulimia. Statements descriptive of binge-eating disorder include those referencing eating rapidly, in large amounts, and feeling uncomfortably full and emotionally bad following the binge. Finally, the last statement is classically associated with obesity, but several of the previous statements may be applicable to an obese client as well, such as those that describe binge-eating disorder.

Goals

Goals are broad statements describing *what you and the client would like the result of therapy to be*. One statement may suffice, but more than one can be used in the treatment plan. Examples of common goal statements for eating disorders and obesity are the following:

➤ Restore normal eating patterns, healthy weight maintenance, and a realistic appraisal of body size.

➤ Stabilize medical condition with balanced fluid and electrolytes, resuming patterns of food intake that will sustain life and gain weight to a normal level.

➤ Terminate the pattern of binge eating and purging behavior with a return to eating normal amounts of nutritious foods.

➤ Terminate overeating and implement lifestyle changes that lead to weight loss and improved health.

➤ Develop healthy cognitive patterns and beliefs about self that lead to positive identity and prevent a relapse of the eating disorder.

For our client with anorexia, we might select a statement like "Restore normal eating patterns, healthy weight maintenance, and a realistic appraisal of body size." For our client with obesity issues, we might select "Terminate overeating and implement lifestyle changes that lead to weight loss and improved health." Other statements could apply to bulimia, and new ones could be added based on what you and your client want to accomplish.

Objectives and Interventions

Objectives are statements that describe *small, observable steps the client must achieve* toward attaining the goal of successful treatment. Intervention statements describe the *actions taken by the therapist* to assist the client in achieving his/her objectives. Each objective must be paired with at least one intervention.

Assessment

All approaches to quality treatment start with a thorough assessment of the nature and history of the client's presenting problems. EST approaches rely on a thorough psychosocial assessment of the nature, history, and severity of the problem as experienced by the client. The first short-term objective and coordinated interventions examine the history of the client's eating pattern, self-perception of body image, personal and interpersonal triggers to problematic eating, and actual weight. The second objective and its two interventions are focused on interviewing for unhealthy use of weight control measures, such as self-induced vomiting, and nonpurging compensatory behaviors, such as fasting and excessive exercise.

Psychological testing or objectives measures may be used as part of the overall assessment of the eating disorder, and then referrals should be made to a physician to rule out possible medical etiologies and assess for any medical effects of the eating disorder or obesity. A nutritional evaluation and possible nutritional rehabilitation may be indicated, particularly in the case of anorexia. A dental exam may be indicated if purging behaviors are used by the client.

Objective 7 could be selected for the client's treatment plan if a psychiatric evaluation is in order to assess the need for psychotropic medications as an adjunct to the treatment. Finally, objective 8 describes the possible need for medical or psychiatric hospitalization if it is determined through assessment that the client's health is severely compromised by the eating disorder or if a significant psychiatric condition, such as a severe mood disorder, is also present.

Table 5.1 contains examples of assessment objectives and interventions for eating disorders and obesity.

Table 5.1   Assessment Objectives and Interventions

Objectives	Interventions
1. Honestly describe the pattern of eating, including types, amounts, and frequency of food restricted, consumed, or hoarded.	1. Establish rapport with the client toward building a therapeutic alliance. 2. Assess the historical course of the disorder, including the amount, type, and pattern of the client's food intake (e.g., too little food, too much food, binge eating, or hoarding food); perceived personal and interpersonal triggers and personal goals. 3. Compare the client's calorie consumption with an average adult rate of 1,900 (for women) to 2,500 (for men) calories per day to determine over- or undereating. 4. Assess the client for minimization and denial of the eating disorder behavior and related distorted thinking and self-perception of body image. 5. Measure the client's weight and begin a chart/graph for ongoing recording of weight changes during treatment.
2. Describe any regular use of unhealthy weight control behaviors.	1. Assess for the presence of self-induced vomiting behavior by the client to purge himself/herself of calorie intake; monitor on an ongoing basis. 2. Assess for nonpurging compensatory behaviors by the client, such as misuse of laxatives, diuretics, enemas, or other medications; fasting; or excessive exercise; monitor on an ongoing basis.
3. Complete psychological testing or objective questionnaires for assessing eating disorders.	1. Administer psychological instruments to the client designed to objectively assess eating disorders (e.g., Eating Inventory by Stunkard and Messick; Stirling Eating Disorder Scales by Williams and Power; or Eating Disorders Inventory-3 [EDI-3] by Garner); give the client feedback regarding the results of the assessment; readminister tests as needed to assess treatment outcome.
4. Cooperate with a complete medical evaluation.	1. Refer the client to a nutritionist who is experienced in eating disorders for an assessment of nutritional rehabilitation; coordinate recommendations into the care plan.
5. Cooperate with a nutritional evaluation.	1. Refer the client to a physician for a medical evaluation to assess negative consequences of failure to maintain adequate body weight and overuse of compensatory behaviors; stay in close consultation with the physician as to the client's medical condition.
6. Cooperate with a dental exam.	1. Refer the client to a dentist for a dental exam to assess the possible damage to teeth from purging behaviors.
7. Cooperate with an evaluation by a physician for psychotropic medication and, if indicated, take medications as prescribed.	1. Assess the client's need for psychotropic medications (e.g., SSRIs); arrange for a physician to evaluate for and then prescribe psychotropic medications, if indicated. 2. Monitor the client's psychotropic medication prescription compliance, effectiveness, and side effects.

Objectives	Interventions
8. Cooperate with admission to inpatient treatment, if indicated.	1. Refer the client for hospitalization, as necessary, if his/her weight loss becomes severe and physical health is jeopardized, or if he/she is severely depressed or suicidal.

Psychoeducation

A typical feature of many ESTs for eating disorders or obesity is initial and ongoing psychoeducation. A common emphasis is helping the client learn about eating disorders or obesity, the treatment, and its rationale. Books or other reading material are often recommended to the client to supplement psychoeducation done in session. It is important to instill hope in the client and have her or him on board as a partner in the treatment process. With ESTs, discussing their demonstrated efficacy with the client can facilitate this hope and cooperation. Objectives nine and ten focus on the client's task of gaining an understanding of the development of his/her condition and the treatment approaches that will be used. The therapist discusses sociocultural pressures that encourage maladaptive eating patterns and provides a rationale for the treatment approach being used. Some reading material may be assigned to aid in educating the client.

Key Points

COMMON EMPHASES OF INITIAL PSYCHOEDUCATION INCLUDE:
1. Teaching the client about the nature and etiology of the diagnosed condition.
2. Informing the client of treatment options, including their research support.
3. Explaining the rationale behind the treatment approach that will be used.
4. Utilizing reading assignments as homework, if needed, to facilitate understanding of psychoeducational goals.

Table 5.2 contains examples of psychoeducational objectives and interventions for eating disorders and obesity.

Table 5.2 Psychoeducation Objectives and Interventions

Objectives	Interventions
9. Verbalize an accurate understanding of how eating disorders develop.	1. Discuss with the client a model of eating disorders development that includes concepts such as sociocultural pressures to be thin, vulnerability in some individuals to overvalue body shape and size in determining self-image, maladaptive eating habits (e.g., fasting, binging, overeating), maladaptive compensatory weight management behaviors (e.g., purging), and resultant feelings of low self-esteem (see *Overcoming Binge Eating* by Fairburn).

(continued)

Objectives	Interventions
10. Verbalize an understanding of the rationale and goals of treatment.	1. Discuss a rationale for treatment that includes using cognitive and behavioral procedures to break the cycle of thinking and behaving that promotes poor self-image, uncontrolled eating, and unhealthy compensatory actions while building physical and mental health-promoting eating practices.
	2. Assign the client to read psychoeducational chapters of books or treatment manuals on the development and treatment of eating disorders or obesity (e.g., *Overcoming Binge Eating* by Fairburn; or *The LEARN Manual* by Brownell for weight loss).

Assessment/Psychoeducation Review

1. What purposes can psychoeducation serve in therapy?
2. What are common emphases of initial psychoeducation?

Assessment/Psychoeducation Review Test Question

1. At what point in therapy is psychoeducation conducted?

   A. At the end of therapy
   B. During the assessment phase
   C. During the initial treatment session
   D. Throughout therapy

Family-Based Treatment for Anorexia

Objective number eleven and its three associated interventions summarize the family-based therapy (FBT) treatment approach for our treatment plan. Phase 1 focuses on taking a history of the eating disorder, clarifying that the parents will be in charge of weight restoration of the client, establishing healthy weight goals, and asking the family to participate in the family meal in session. In Phase 2 of this treatment, weight continues to be closely monitored. Control over eating is gradually turned over to the adolescent client as normal eating patterns emerge. Finally, in Phase 3, the focus is on consolidating and reinforcing the new stabilized eating patterns and weight gain. Adolescent developmental issues are addressed, and problem-solving and relapse prevention skills are also typically taught.

Key Points

THREE PHASES OF FBT FOR ANOREXIA

PHASE 1

- Parents are placed in charge of the nutritional rehabilitation and weight restoration.
- "The family meal" serves as an arena for assessment and intervention.
- The adolescent's autonomy in other life areas, such as school and social domains, is kept intact.

PHASE 2

- Control over eating is shifted to the adolescent, based on sufficient patient weight gain.
- There should be evidence of eating without undue prompting or struggle with parents.
- Parents should feel empowered.
- Patient should feel relief that he or she can manage the feeding process.

PHASE 3

- Families are prepared for termination of therapy.
- Important adolescent issues are reviewed.
- Use of problem solving is taught.
- Possible future issues are planned for.
- Use of therapy skills to address them is reviewed.

Table 5.3 contains examples of a FBT objective and interventions for anorexia nervosa.

Table 5.3   Family-Based Treatment Objective and Interventions

Objective	Interventions
11. Parents and adolescent with anorexia agree to participate in all three phases of family-based treatment of anorexia through 20 sessions over 12 months.	1. Begin Phase 1 (sessions 1–10) of family-based treatment by confirming with the family their intent to participate and strictly adhere to the treatment plan, taking a history of the eating disorder, clarifying that the parents will be in charge of weight restoration of the client, establishing healthy weight goals, and asking the family to participate in the family meal in session; establish with the parents and a physician a minimum daily caloric intake for the client and focus them on meal planning; consult with a physician and/or nutritionist if fluids and electrolytes need monitoring because of the adolescent's poor nutritional habits. 2. In Phase 2 (sessions 11–16), continue to closely monitor weight gain and physician/nutritionist reports regarding health status; gradually return control over eating decisions back to the adolescent as the acute starvation is resolved and portions consumed are nearing what is normally expected and weight gain in demonstrated. 3. In Phase 3 (sessions 17–20), review and reinforce progress and weight gain; focus on adolescent development issues; teach and rehearse problem-solving and relapse prevention skills.

Demonstration Vignette

Family-Based Treatment for Anorexia

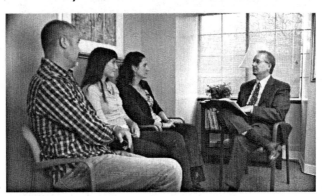

Here we present the transcript of the dialogue depicted in the Family-Based Treatment therapy vignette.

Therapist: How have things been since our last session?

Dad: I think they've been a lot better.

Therapist: How so?

Dad: Well, Danielle has worked her way off her plateau, and she's gained a few more pounds.

Therapist: Joan, what's your impression?

Mom: The same. A few weeks ago I didn't think she was getting enough calories, but over the past few weeks she's been taking bigger portions, and without us having to ask her to.

Therapist: You've been monitoring her eating and calorie intake closely?

Mom: Oh yes.

Therapist: Good. You too, Tom?

Dad: Yeah. We've been giving Danielle a little more choice in what and how much she eats, and she's been eating well.

Therapist: Good! I'm glad to hear that. So, why did you decide to start giving Danielle more choice?

Mom: Well, Danielle asked us to, but also because she's doing better. She sometimes gives us that look, you know, like we're prison guards watching the prisoner.

Therapist: Do you feel like a prisoner, Danielle?

Danielle: Sometimes. It's like, I don't know, I just feel like they think I'm not going to do what I'm supposed to—like they don't trust me.

Therapist: Is that your concern, you don't trust her?

Dad: No, we just want her to be able to succeed.

Mom: Yeah, we just don't want this thing to take control again. It's not her, it's the anorexia.

Therapist: How do you feel about that, Danielle?

Danielle: I know that. It's just I feel like I can do this now. I don't need them to watch everything I do.

Therapist: Okay. Well, you know, this treatment program moves in phases. In the beginning, the parents take the primary responsibility for ensuring that eating patterns are stable and sufficient to allow weight to be gained. That's because of the health risks involved. But at

	some point, we make the transition to having Danielle assume more of that responsibility again. Danielle, it sounds like you think you are ready to begin that.
Danielle:	I do.
Therapist:	So what makes you think so?
Danielle:	Well, I think I'm doing well. I mean the doctor said so.
Therapist:	That's good. I saw that in the doctor's report. Besides the doctor telling you your health is improving, what have you noticed in *yourself* that makes you feel you're ready?
Danielle:	Well, I'm eating larger portions. I'm doing that myself. And I'm taking my calcium every day. I didn't like hearing about how my bones could get that brittle and that it's going to take awhile for them to get strong again.
Therapist:	You're more concerned with the health risks, and that's motivating you more than it used to?
Danielle:	Yeah. I always kind of knew about them, but I guess when it's actually happened to me it was different. I'm feeling better, and I can see it's because I'm eating.
Therapist:	That's different than when you first started treatment?
Danielle:	Yes. When I first heard that I was gaining weight, it was kind of scary, but after a while it didn't bother me as much.
Therapist:	Is it still a struggle?
Danielle:	Not like it used to be. I think I'm doing a lot better just focusing on getting healthier and getting my life back. I feel like I'm ready to get my life back.
Therapist:	I can see that. So how do you guys feel about handing over some of this responsibility to Danielle? Are you ready? Do you think she's ready?
Mom:	I think so. I still want to know how she's doing.
Dad:	I'm thinking we can try it.
Therapist:	So how can we hand some of this responsibility back to Danielle and also feel assured that she's continuing her success?
Dad:	What about the doctor's report? I mean, if they continue to be good, then we know she must be doing well. If not, I guess we just go back to what we were doing.
Therapist:	Joan, how does that strike you?
Mom:	That sounds good.
Therapist:	Danielle, do you have a problem with the plan your Mom and Dad are suggesting?—Let you take control over what and how much you eat, use the doctor's report, and talk here?
Danielle:	No, I know I can do it.
Therapist:	Okay, good. Let's just talk more specifically about what this eating pattern will look like over the next week and the targets we'd like to see in the doctor's report. [Everyone nods in agreement.]

Critique of the Family-Based Treatment Demonstration Vignette

The following points were made in the critique:

a. Session starts with reviewing how parents have been in control in Phase 1 of this treatment.

b. Transition to Phase 2 is being considered, with the therapist getting the perspective of all the family members and allowing them to make the decision about whether everyone is comfortable with the change to the client being more in control of her eating.

c. If weight loss happens, an immediate return to Phase 1 is in order.

d. The specifics of what Phase 2 will be like for the client and the parents are drawn out.

e. The criteria for success in Stage 2 are specified, including the physician's evaluation role.

f. It is important to keep the family unit working together on the problem, accepting joint responsibility and clearly communicating with each other.

Additional points that could be made:

a. The therapist uses reflection effectively to draw out the client's thoughts and feelings.

b. The client's motivation for change is drawn out of her.

c. It is noteworthy that no fears of weight gain were made by the client, which is a positive sign of improvement.

Comments you would like to make:

_____

_____

_____

_____

Homework: Perhaps as part of the assessment in Phase 1 of Family-Based Treatment, you might assign "Reality: Food Intake, Weight, Thoughts, and Feelings" (*Adolescent Psychotherapy Homework Planner*, 2nd ed., by Jongsma, Peterson, & McInnis) to get the client to face the facts of what and how much has been eaten and how eating sets off a cognitive chain reaction that leads to irrational fear and dysfunctional weight control behaviors. Also, "Plan and Eat a Meal" (*Adolescent Psychotherapy Homework Planner II*, by Jongsma, Peterson, & McInnis) fits right into the practice of having the family plan a meal and bring it to a therapy session to eat together. The exercise encourages the family to increase levity and enjoyment during the meal to offset the usual stress and conflict that accompanies mealtime when an eating disorder invades the family (see www.wiley.com/go/edowb).

Family–Based Treatment Review

1. What are primary emphases within each of the three phases of FBT for anorexia nervosa?

Family-Based Treatment Review Test Question

1. Which of the following is *not* characteristic of the first phase of family-based treatment for anorexia nervosa?

    A. Control over eating is given to the adolescent patient.
    B. Parents are placed in charge of the nutritional rehabilitation and weight restoration of their adolescent child.
    C. The family eats some meals in therapy while the therapist assesses interactions.
    D. The seriousness of the disorder is conveyed.

Cognitive-Behavioral Therapy for Bulimia

Cognitive-Behavioral Therapy (CBT) has been identified as a research-supported treatment for late adolescents and adults with bulimia. To represent this approach, we have written objective twelve for the client to achieve and its six integrated interventions for the therapist to implement. Intervention one for this objective focuses on psychoeducation and self-monitoring of relevant features of bulimia. A regular pattern of eating is established. The therapeutic interventions in the second phase of CBT for bulimia lean heavily on teaching problem solving and doing cognitive restructuring to identify, challenge, and replace negative cognitive messages that mediate feelings and actions leading to maladaptive eating and weight control practices. Homework assignments may be used in any of these phases to reinforce

---

Key Points

THREE PHASES OF CBT TREATMENT FOR BULIMIA NERVOSA
PHASE 1

- Psychoeducation on adverse effects of binging, purging, extreme dieting
- Encourages regular pattern of eating and reasonable weight monitoring frequency
- Stimulus control procedures applied to eating times and places, food shopping times
- Self-control strategies address healthy alternative activities to binging

PHASE 2

- Uses cognitive restructuring targeting dieting, shape, and weight concerns
- Problem solving used to manage causes of stress

PHASE 3

- Develops a maintenance plan
- Implements relapse prevention strategies

the achievement of the client objective. The final phase of CBT focuses on strengthening skills and gains made in therapy as well as relapse prevention. Intervention number three captures these emphases.

Table 5.4 contains examples of a Cognitive-Behavioral Therapy objective and interventions for bulimia nervosa.

Table 5.4   Cognitive–Behavioral Therapy Objective and Interventions

Objective	Interventions
12. Participate in cognitive-behavioral therapy to identify, challenge, and replace self-talk and beliefs that promote the bulimia.	1. Conduct Phase 1 of cognitive-behavioral therapy: focusing the client on psychoeducation regarding the adverse effects of binging and purging, assigning self-monitoring of weight and eating patterns, and establishing a regular pattern of eating (use "A Reality Journal: Food, Weight, Thoughts, and Feelings" in the *Adult Psychotherapy Homework Planner*, 2nd ed., by Jongsma or "Daily Record of Dysfunctional Thoughts" in *Cognitive Therapy of Depression* by Beck, Rush, Shaw, & Emery); process the journal material.
	2. In Phase 2 of CBT, shift the focus to eliminating dieting, reducing weight and body image concerns, teaching problem solving, and doing cognitive restructuring to identify, challenge, and replace negative cognitive messages that mediate feelings and actions leading to maladaptive eating and weight control practices (consider assigning "Fears Beneath the Eating Disorder" from the *Adolescent Psychotherapy Homework Planner*, 2nd ed., by Jongsma, Peterson, and McInnis.)
	3. In Phase 3 of CBT, assist the client in developing a maintenance and relapse prevention plan, including self-monitoring of eating and binge triggers, continuing to use problem solving and cognitive restructuring, and setting short-term goals to stay on track.

Demonstration Vignette

Cognitive-Behavioral Therapy for Bulimia

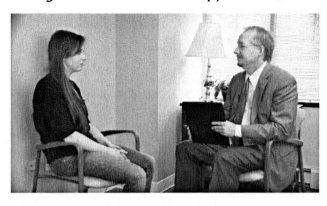

Here we present the transcript of the dialogue depicted in the Cognitive-Behavioral Therapy vignette.

Therapist: So given what we've discussed and what you've read, what's your take on this cycle?

Client: Well, it seems like when I try dieting it eventually makes me want to binge. Then I feel bad, like I'm going to gain weight, so I purge. Then it just repeats over and over.

Therapist: And how do you feel after purging?

Client: Well, honestly, I feel good and bad.

Therapist: How so?

Client: Well, good in that I feel like I won't gain weight, but bad because, well, I feel like I can't control myself.

Therapist: So, by restricting your diet, it actually drives your urge to binge. Then binging leads to fears of gaining weight and makes you want to purge. You feel better temporarily, but then you start to feel guilty—like you don't feel in control. And then the cycle repeats itself the next time around.

Client: Yeah. That sounds like me.

Therapist: Binging does this to everyone. Does it make sense to you that if you can break this cycle, it'll help you reach your goals?

Client: Yeah, but I haven't been able to.

Therapist: I understand. Let's talk about our first step, regulating when you eat.

Client: Okay, I understand about trying to get on a regular eating pattern. But if I stop skipping meals to help reduce the urge to binge, won't I just gain a bunch of weight?

Therapist: Well, remember, we agreed that our first goal is to reduce the binging and purging. Having said that, most people don't gain a bunch of weight when they make this transition. In fact, most find that their weight fluctuates more, down and up, when they're not on a regular schedule.

Client: Really?

Therapist: Yeah, part of this is because we are regulating *when* you eat, not how much, or what you eat. Establishing a regular pattern reduces urges to binge, so your overall calories don't necessarily have to be more. It depends on the type of meals and snacks you have.

Client: I see. I guess I'm worrying about the weight issue again, huh? It's hard to just weigh myself once a week.

Therapist: I know. Do you mind if we talk a little more about that—weight, health, and how these two things relate to one another. Then maybe we can start to look at what your meals and snacks could be, when and where you are going to eat, and the like. Does that sound okay?

Client: Okay.

Client: I know I need to get used to the full feeling being normal, and not a sign that I've overeaten. That's hard.

Therapist: What's hardest about it for you?

Client: The urges—how to deal with them.

Therapist: Okay, let's talk about that. One of the first things to know in coping with urges is that if you can ride them out some, they will decrease. The urges get weaker.

Client: I read that in the workbook. I guess I've never really waited to see, but the workbook did have a graph.

(continued)

Therapist: That's right. [Therapist shows client a piece of paper with a wave shape on it.] The urge actually does something like this: it does go up to a point, but then it comes down. Our goal is to get past that hump.

Client: It looks like a wave.

Therapist: Exactly. That's why some people call this "surfing the urge."

Client: Surfing the urge, huh? I guess I've never surfed before. [smiles]

Therapist: Let's talk about "how to surf" then. What do you say?

Client: All right.

Therapist: So you're worried about this thing coming up Friday night?

Client: Yeah. I'm sure some people are going to bring snacks and stuff, and I don't want to, you know, fall off the wagon.

Therapist: Okay, so let's problem-solve like we've done with the others. First, let's define the problem specifically. We know the situation, so what's your goal?

Client: I don't want to overeat snacks at the party, I suppose.

Therapist: That's good. That's specific: "I want to prevent myself from overeating snacks at the party." Let's move to options that might help us do this. Can you think of any?

Client: I was thinking I would take my own snack and limit the amount I eat that way.

Therapist: Just eat what you bring?

Client: Yeah. If anyone asks, I could just say my snack sits better with me or something.

Therapist: Okay, we'll wait to evaluate that option. Other options?

Client: I was thinking of taking some sugar-free tea with me, to keep me satisfied, so I don't feel like drinking stuff that will tempt me to purge.

Therapist: Okay. Let's look at some more options, and then we'll evaluate the pros and cons of them all.

Critique of the Cognitive–Behavioral Therapy Demonstration Vignette

The following points were made in the critique:

a. Therapist makes good use of psychoeducation throughout the session, giving the client sound factual information regarding eating, diet, and weight.

b. Therapist uses reflective listening techniques effectively along with summarizing to clarify cycles of bulimia.

c. Coping skills are taught to the client to help her "surf the urge."

d. The specifics of a high-risk situation for binging are clarified, and then problem-solving techniques are applied to the issue.

e. Therapist is effective at drawing options out of the client for coping with the high-risk eating situation.

f. The session demonstrates multiple CBT techniques being applied: psychoeducation, cognitive restructuring, coping skills, and problem solving.

Additional points that could be made:

a. The therapist is working to get the client to accept and develop regular eating patterns, and pointing out her thoughts about not skipping meals triggers fears of weight gain.

Comments you would like to make:

_____

_____

_____

_____

    Homework: Table 5.4 lists the objectives and interventions for CBT for bulimia. Three homework exercises are included there: "A Reality Journal: Food, Weight, Thoughts and Feelings," "Fears Beneath the Eating Disorder" (*Adult Psychotherapy Homework Planner*, 2nd ed., by Jongsma), and "Daily Record of Dysfunctional Thoughts" (*Cognitive Therapy of Depression* by Beck, Rush, Shaw, & Emery). Distorted self-talk about the body is addressed in "Body Image" (*Adolescent Psychotherapy Homework Planner, 2nd ed.*, by Jongsma, Peterson, & McInnis) and in "What Am I Thinking?" (*Group Therapy Homework Planner* by Bevilaqua). An additional assignment that focuses on helping the client become aware of common cognitive distortions and how they influence emotions is "Negative Thoughts Trigger Negative Emotions" (*Adult Psychotherapy Homework Planner*, 2nd ed., by Jongsma). (See www.wiley.com/go/edowb.)

Cognitive-Behavioral Therapy Review

    1. What are primary emphases of CBT for bulimia nervosa?

Cognitive-Behavioral Therapy Review Test Question

    1. Which of the following is a primary focus of cognitive-behavioral therapy (CBT) for bulimia nervosa (BN)?

        A. How bulimia is an expression of a fixation from an earlier stage of development

        B. How early attachment problems with primary caregivers have made the client vulnerable to bulimic acting out

        C. How interpersonal issues such as disputes with parents and grief underlie the bulimia

        D. How the current cycle of binging, purging, and concerns about body weight and shape operate in a cycle to maintain the disorder

Interpersonal Therapy

Objective thirteen describes the client objective for the Interpersonal Therapy (IPT) approach. Phase 1 of this therapy involves a thorough assessment of the eating disorder as well as important past and present interpersonal relationships. The therapist takes the lead in doing this Interpersonal Inventory, and assesses interpersonal issues such as disputes, role transition conflicts, unresolved grief, and interpersonal deficits. In the second phase of treatment, the client takes the lead by talking freely about the identified problem area or areas, exploring alternative ways to view the problem and resolve it. The final phase focuses on consolidating and reinforcing the interpersonal gains made and developing a relapse prevention plan.

Key Points

THREE PHASES OF IPT FOR BULIMIA
PHASE 1: THERAPIST LEADS

- Assessment of bulimia
- Taking Interpersonal Inventory of past and present relationships

PHASE 2: CLIENT LEADS

- Themes: role disputes, role transitions, interpersonal deficits, unresolved grief
- Client explores change in interpersonal problems
- Nondirective in nature
- Role-play and problem solving used

PHASE 3

- Consolidate gains
- Relapse prevention

Table 5.5 contains examples of an Interpersonal Therapy objective and interventions for bulimia nervosa.

Table 5.5   Interpersonal Therapy Objective and Interventions

Objective	Interventions
13. Discuss important people in your life, past and present, and describe the quality, good and bad, of those relationships.	1. In Phase 1 of Interpersonal Therapy (IPT), assess the client's Interpersonal Inventory of important past and present relationships, highlighting themes that may be supporting the bulimia (e.g., interpersonal disputes, role transition conflict, unresolved grief, and/or interpersonal deficits).
	2. In Phase 2 of IPT, encourage the client to take the lead in facilitating change in the interpersonal arena by keeping him/her focused on talking about the problem areas, clarifying issues, and encouraging change.
	3. In Phase 3 of IPT, focus the client on gains made in the interpersonal realm and on developing a bulimia relapse prevention plan.

Demonstration Vignette
Interpersonal Therapy for Bulimia

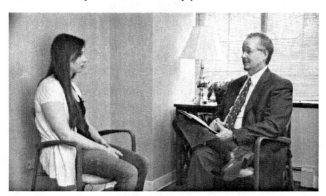

Here we present the transcript of the dialogue depicted in the Interpersonal Therapy vignette.

Therapist: I just want to explain the nature of this therapy so that you have a good sense of what to expect.

Client: Okay.

Therapist: It's helpful to think of our therapy as having two distinct phases. The first phase, which may take a few sessions, is for information gathering. I want to learn about the eating problem, from when it began until now. I also want to learn about important past and present relationships. I'll take the lead in this phase by asking you questions. Your role is to just answer and discuss the issues with me the best you can. When I have a sufficient understanding of these things, you and I will discuss and come to an agreement on which issue or issues we will focus on for the rest of the therapy. Does that sound okay to you?

Client: It sounds okay.

Therapist: All right, after this information-gathering phase, the nature of the therapy will change. Instead of me asking you questions and you answering them, you'll take more of the lead by talking about the issue or issues we agreed to focus on. You can talk about whatever you like regarding the issue you select. I may have questions or comments to get the ball rolling, but for the most part you are just expected to explore your thoughts and feelings about the issue and also be open to possibly trying new ways of approaching them. Doing this is intended to increase your understanding of the issues and may lead to some positive changes. Are you willing to try that?

Client: I can try. I'm not used to talking about this stuff, but I'm here to get better, so I'll try.

Therapist: Very good. That's all that's asked. Ready to get started?

Client: Sure.

Therapist: Okay, let's start with the eating problem. Looking back, when did this start for you?

Client: I guess I was about 11 years old when I first heard of bulimia, but I didn't try it until I was 14.

Therapist: In our last session you mentioned that your parents were divorced when you were 12, and you stayed with your mother?

Client: Yeah, I lived with my mom, but we moved to a new house and I went to a new school.

(continued)

Therapist:	What was that like for you?
Client:	I hated it.
Therapist:	What about it did you hate?
Client:	Well, I lost all my old friends, and I was the "new kid," you know? There were already all these cliques established. I had to eat lunch by myself.
Therapist:	You felt lonely?
Client:	Oh yeah. Plus, the people at that school were mean. Some of the popular girls would make fun of the way I looked, my clothes. They'd call me "plain," "fat," say things like, "Oh my gosh, look at that dress!" Stuff like that.
Therapist:	How do you recall feeling about that at the time?
Client:	Like I just wanted to get out of there. Go back to my old school, my old friends.
Therapist:	We have been talking about your moving and the struggles of attending a new school.
Client:	I guess I started to doubt myself back then. My Dad had left us. I felt like he must not have loved me.
Therapist:	He left because he didn't love you?
Client:	No, I guess not. He and Mom weren't happy. But he left, and then he got remarried.
Therapist:	You felt abandoned?
Client:	Kind of. [Therapist waits while patient is silent for about 5 seconds.] I mean I know that just because he got remarried doesn't mean he didn't love me, but it felt that way.
Therapist:	At that time you saw it as him not loving you, but you now see that there may have been other reasons why he remarried?
Client:	Yeah. I mean, he was happier. But I guess I was feeling like, I don't know, like he was happier without me.
Therapist:	You thought your absence and not his wife's presence was what was making him look happier?
Client:	I guess so. I know that's not why, but I guess I was feeling that way—rejected.
Therapist:	You started to doubt yourself because at the time you didn't fully understand why your Dad was doing what he was doing—you thought it was because something was wrong with you, that he was rejecting you, and it made him happier?
Client:	I guess so. I've never really talked with my Dad about this.
Therapist:	You're thinking about doing that?
Client:	Maybe it's time.

Critique of the Interpersonal Therapy Demonstration Vignette

The following points were made in the critique:

a. The therapist provides structure in explaining the changing roles that will be taken by himself and the client as they move from Phase 1 to Phase 2.

b. In Phase 1, the therapist is asking questions and taking the lead in doing an Interpersonal Inventory.

c. In Phase 2, the therapist is using reflective listening techniques to help the client clarify thoughts and feelings about interpersonal relationships.

d. Client is developing some insight about her father, but therapist leaves it up to the client as to whether she will decide to talk to her father about whether she had anything to do with his decision to divorce her mother.

e. Role-play may be used to facilitate her talk with her dad.

Additional points that could be made:

a. It is noteworthy that the therapist does not make a direct connection (interpretation) between the client's interpersonal issues with her father and her development of bulimia. That is not his role in IPT.

b. Therapist did not mention Phase 3 in which a relapse prevention plan will be created.

Comments you would like to make:

_____

_____

_____

_____

Homework: Although the vignette emphasizes the nondirective, reflective listening nature of Phase 2 of IPT, some cognitive-behavioral techniques are also used to assist in resolving interpersonal disputes. Problem-solving skills may be applied first through didactic, then role-play, and then assigned to be applied to actual life relationships. The exercise "Applying Problem-Solving to Interpersonal Conflict" (*Adult Psychotherapy Homework Planner*, 2nd ed., by Jongsma) is consistent with this IPT approach may be useful to the therapeutic process (see www.wiley.com/go/edowb).

Interpersonal Therapy Review

1. How is IPT for bulimia nervosa conducted and what are its emphases?

Interpersonal Therapy Review Test Question

1. Which of the following best characterizes an emphasis of the first phase of interpersonal therapy (IPT) for bulimia nervosa?

   A. Assessing important past and present relationships
   B. Addressing grief
   C. Addressing role transitions
   D. Training interpersonal skills

Behavioral Weight Loss Treatments

Behavioral Weight Loss (BWL) treatments are a set of identified research-supported treatments for obesity. The most studied of these treatments is the LEARN program, which emphasizes change in Lifestyle, Exercise, Attitudes, Relationships, and Nutrition. To integrate this approach into our treatment plan, we suggest statements such as our objective number fourteen, which refers to the implementation of these five emphases of the program. The first intervention refers to psychoeducation to introduce and clarify the five facets of LEARN. The second intervention describes the heart of the LEARN approach, in which the client and therapist work their way through the program's emphases to establish new eating patterns through overall behavior change.

Key Points

CHARACTERISTICS OF BEHAVIORAL WEIGHT LOSS PROGRAMS SUCH AS **LEARN:**

- Sets reasonable expectations and weight goals
- Teaches healthy nutrition
- Prescribes moderation in food choice
- Encourages small changes in daily lifestyle activity
- Teaches cognitive restructuring
- Teaches behavioral skills such as communication, problem solving, and relapse prevention

---

Table 5.6 contains examples of a LEARN program objective and interventions for obesity treatment.

Table 5.6   LEARN Program Objective and Interventions

Objective	Interventions
14. Follow through on implementing the five aspects of the LEARN program to achieve weight loss.	1. Assign the client to read the LEARN Manual and then review the five aspects of the program that will be emphasized over the next 12 weeks. 2. In weekly sessions, systematically work through the five aspects of the LEARN program manual (Lifestyle, Exercise, Attitudes, Relationships, and Nutrition), applying each component to the client's life to establish new behavioral patterns designed to achieve weight loss.

Demonstration Vignette
LEARN Program for Obesity

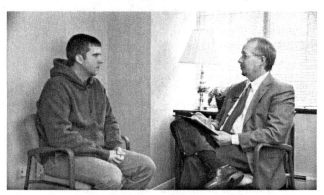

Here we present the transcript of the dialogue depicted in the LEARN program therapy vignette.

Therapist: Bob, I know you have done some reading by now about the LEARN weight management program. So you know that the central tenet of the program is that you must develop new habits and make them a permanent part of your new life. It's not a diet program—it's a lifestyle change program. The focus is on behavior change that leads to weight loss. And because much of our behavior stems from the way we think and make decisions, we also want to look at those thinking patterns and see if they are helping us with our behavior change goals.

Client: Yeah, I read the introduction of the manual and it makes sense.

Therapist: Good. Why don't we take a quick look at the five aspects of the LEARN program and introduce how they might apply to your life. The L of the LEARN acronym stands for Lifestyle. What lifestyle changes, your day-to-day activities, do you see for yourself to bring about your weight loss?

Client: Well, I have to stay away from sweets and soda. I get a lot of unnecessary calories right there.

Therapist: All right. That's a good insight. So one thing the program will suggest is to eliminate high-calorie foods from the house or from easy access. Replacing sweet snacks with healthy snacks is another. We'll talk more about that later.

Client: I also eat when I'm not hungry. That has to change.

Therapist: Perfect. Learning skills to cope with those moments is part of this too. We can talk about how to use things like distracting activities and enforced eating delays that might help you achieve this goal.

So let's move on for now to the second aspect of the program. The E stands for Exercise. What about your physical activity level?

Client: I certainly don't get enough exercise. I play golf once a week and walk the dog around the block, but that's about it.

Therapist: Perhaps we can build on it. This program will encourage you to try to increase activity on a daily basis. So, for example, we may consider increasing your walk around the block to more vigorous daily walking. It will help if you keep a diary of your exercise and perhaps

(continued)

	find a partner to exercise with. Accountability and social support can be beneficial in accomplishing this behavior change.
Client:	I know it would be good for me to get off the couch and be more active.
Therapist:	All right. So the third component of the LEARN program is Attitude change. Do you see a need for this for yourself?
Client:	I'm not sure what it means.
Therapist:	One aspect of attitude is focused on thinking traps that can derail your progress. For example, being too perfectionistic or rigid in your attempt to change your behavior is an attitude issue—"If I'm not perfect, I've failed." Setting realistic goals, using positive, confident self-talk rather than pessimistic, discouraging self-talk is another part this. Does that help you?
Client:	Yeah, I see. I've tended to get easily discouraged in the past—when things got off track. So this is an area that I need some help.
Therapist:	Excellent. Your openness to change and readiness to change is likely to help you. Now the fourth letter in our acronym is R for Relationship resources. What thoughts do you have about this, Bob?
Client:	Well, my wife has been after me for years to get serious about weight loss, so I'm sure she'll encourage me.
Therapist:	Okay. Telling friends and family of your lifestyle change and asking them to support you is strongly encouraged in this program.
	Now, the final component of the LEARN program is N for Nutrition. Do you have a solid understanding of healthy nutrition, Bob?
Client:	Oh, I understand the five major food groups, but that's about it. I sure don't eat the recommended servings.
Therapist:	The program does teach you the recommended number of servings for the food groups. It also teaches you to be aware of calorie content, serving size, fat content, and a balanced diet. Changing eating behaviors is likely to be more successful when you have sound nutritional information.
Client:	I know I have to make some lifestyle changes to maintain any weight loss, or I'll just regain it like I've done before.
Therapist:	Exactly. This program consists of approximately 12 weekly lessons that are summarized in the manual you've started reading. We'll be following this pretty closely over the next three months, so reading will help you stay on top of things.
Client:	I think I'm ready to get started.

Critique of the LEARN Program Demonstration Vignette

The following points were made in the critique:

a. This is an overview of LEARN and includes assessment as well as psychoeducation.

b. The client is nicely brought into the discussion by asking for his reaction, input, and application to his life.

c. This can be done in a group format as well, and group member input can be solicited by the leader.

d. The therapist makes good use of examples to clarify and explain concepts and components.

e. This is another example of integrating homework into the session, as the client has been given a LEARN reading assignment before this session.

Additional points that could be made:

a. Therapist stresses that LEARN is not a diet but a lifestyle and behavior change program.

b. A cognitive restructuring aspect is introduced when the therapist talks about the need for positive self-talk during the Attitude component explanation.

Comments you would like to make:

_____
_____
_____
_____

Homework: These four homework exercises (*Group Therapy Homework Planner* by Bevilaqua) may fit into various steps in the LEARN program: "Am I Hungry?" helps clients recognize when they are feeling physically hungry and need to eat, as opposed to eating from emotional stress; "I Need to Get Control" uses a cognitive-behavioral approach to help clients understand the link between their thoughts and their eating behavior; "What Am I Thinking?" addresses the types of thinking errors engaged in and the feelings and behavior triggered by them; and "Is It Good Food or Bad Food? Should It Matter That Much?" is designed to help clients break away from rigid thinking about food and to allow themselves the flexibility and freedom to eat reasonably without feeling badly (see www.wiley.com/go/edowb).

LEARN Program Review

1. What are key emphases of behavioral weight loss programs?

LEARN Program Review Test Question

1. LEARN is the well-studied version of behavioral weight loss treatments. For what does the acronym stand?

   A. Labor, Engage, Act, Ply, and Now

   B. Lifestyle, Exercise, Attitudes, Relationships, and Nutrition

C. Listen, Examine, Analyze, Review, and Note

D. Love, Endear, Adore, Relate, and Nap

Chapter References

Bevilacqua, Louis. (2002). *Group Therapy Homework Planner*. New York: Wiley, 2002.

Jongsma, Arthur E. (2006). *Adult Psychotherapy Homework Planner* (2nd ed.). Hoboken, NJ: Wiley.

Jongsma, Arthur E., L. Mark. Peterson, and William P. McInnis. (2006). Adolescent Psychotherapy Homework Planner (2nd ed.). Hoboken, NJ: Wiley.

6

What Are Common Considerations for Relapse Prevention?

Whether treated pharmacologically or psychologically, eating disorders and obesity are prone to relapse. By their nature, research-supported treatments for anorexia nervosa are relapse preventative. Treatments for bulimia, binge-eating disorder, and obesity also place a heavy emphasis on preventing relapse. Let's look at some common considerations in relapse prevention and how they can be incorporated into your treatment plan.

1. Provide a rationale for relapse prevention that discusses the risk and introduces strategies for preventing it.
   - ➢ One of the first steps in relapse prevention interventions is to provide a *rationale* for them. This typically involves a discussion of the risk for relapse and how using the relapse prevention approach we will outline can lower that risk.

2. Discuss with the client the distinction between a lapse and relapse, associating a lapse with a temporary setback and relapse with a return to a sustained pattern of thinking, feeling, and acting consistent with the eating disorder or obesity.
   - ➢ Another initial step in this relapse prevention approach is to distinguish between a lapse and relapse. A lapse is presented as a temporary setback that may involve, for example, re-experiencing an urge to binge or purge, beginning to restrict one's diet again, or starting to skip exercise sessions after having established a program.
   - ➢ Relapse is described as a return to a more sustained pattern of thinking, feeling, and acting that is characteristic of the previous eating disorder or problem. The rationale for this distinction is that a lapse does not need to develop into a relapse if it can be caught and managed.

3. Identify and rehearse managing high-risk situations for a lapse.
   - ➢ High-risk situations that might make the client vulnerable to a lapse are identified.

> For the high-risk situations identified, the therapist leads the client in a rehearsal of using skills learned in therapy to manage them, such as those involved in surfing urges or asserting oneself with family and friends.

> In addition to using skills learned in therapy to manage high-risk situations, clients are encouraged to use strategies learned in therapy during their day-to-day life to help maintain gains and prevent relapse. Examples include maintaining a regular eating schedule, making self-statements reflecting the new messages gained through cognitive restructuring, and consistently using problem-solving skills to address problems.

5. Develop a coping card, or other memory aid, on which coping strategies and other important information can be kept.

> Sometimes clients benefit from having a coping card or some other reminder of important strategies and information regarding relapse prevention.

6. Schedule periodic maintenance or booster sessions to help the client maintain therapeutic gains and problem-solve challenges.

> Periodic booster sessions of therapy can help reinforce positive changes, problem-solve challenges, and facilitate continued improvement, so clients are invited to periodically revisit therapy for these purposes.

Common Considerations in Relapse Prevention

1. Explain the rationale of relapse prevention interventions
2. Distinguish between lapse and relapse
3. Identify and rehearse managing high-risk situations for a lapse
4. Encourage routine use of skills learned in therapy
5. Consider developing a coping card
6. Schedule periodic booster therapy sessions

Table 6.1   Integrating Relapse Prevention Objectives and Interventions Into the Treatment Plan

Objectives	Interventions
15. Verbalize an understanding of relapse prevention and the difference between a lapse and relapse.	1. Provide a rationale for relapse prevention that discusses the risk and introduces strategies for preventing it. 2. Discuss with the client the distinction between a lapse and relapse, associating a lapse with a temporary setback and relapse with a return to a sustained pattern of thinking, feeling, and behaving that is characteristic of eating disorders and obesity.

(continued)

Objectives	Interventions
16. Identify potential situations that could trigger a lapse and implement strategies to prevent and manage these situations.	1. Reviewing past anxiety-producing situations, assist the client in identifying future situations or circumstances in which lapses could occur. 2. Rehearse with clients the use of strategies learned in therapy to manage high-risk situations (e.g., calming and coping skills); simultaneously encourage clients to integrate skills learned in therapy (e.g., relaxation, cognitive restructuring, problem solving) into their day-to-day life to help maintain gains, prevent relapse, and manage trigger situations. 3. Develop a coping card on which coping strategies and other important information can be kept (e.g., steps in problem solving, positive coping statements, reminders that were helpful to clients during therapy). 4. Schedule periodic maintenance or booster sessions to help clients maintain therapeutic gains and problem-solve challenges.

Chapter Review

1. What are the common considerations in relapse prevention?

Chapter Review Test Question

1. Sam and his therapist are talking about future situations that could challenge him and potentially set him back if he encounters one. They plan to review these encounters and develop a plan for coping with them in common sessions. Which consideration in relapse prevention is being conducted in the current session?

   A. Developing a coping card
   B. Distinguishing between a lapse and relapse
   C. Encouraging the routine use of skills learned in therapy
   D. Identifying high-risk situations for a lapse

Closing Remarks and Resources

As we note on the DVD, it is important to be aware that the research support for any particular EST supports the identified treatment as it was delivered in the studies supporting it. The use of only selected objectives or interventions from ESTs may not be empirically supported.

If you want to incorporate an EST into your treatment plan, it should reflect the major objectives and interventions of the approach. Note that in addition to their primary objectives and interventions, many ESTs have options within them that may or may not be used depending on the client's need (e.g., skills training). Most treatment manuals, books, and other training programs identify the primary objectives and interventions used in the EST.

An existing resource for integrating research-supported treatments into treatment planning is the Practice*Planners*® series[1] of treatment planners. The series contains several books that have integrated goals, objectives, and interventions consistent with those of identified ESTs into treatment plans for several applicable problems and disorders:

➤ *The Severe and Persistent Mental Illness Treatment Planner* (Berghuis, Jongsma, & Bruce)
➤ *The Family Therapy Treatment Planner* (Dattilio, Jongsma, & Davis)
➤ *The Complete Adult Psychotherapy Treatment Planner* (Jongsma, Peterson, & Bruce)
➤ *The Adolescent Psychotherapy Treatment Planner* (Jongsma, Peterson, McInnis, & Bruce)
➤ *The Child Psychotherapy Treatment Planner* (Jongsma, Peterson, McInnis, & Bruce)

---

[1]These books are updated frequently; check with the publisher for the latest editions and for further information about the Practice*Planners*®.

➢ *The Veterans and Active Duty Military Psychotherapy Treatment Planner* (Moore & Jongsma)

➢ *The Addiction Treatment Planner* (Perkinson, Jongsma, & Bruce)

➢ *The Couples Psychotherapy Treatment Planner* (O'Leary, Heyman, & Jongsma)

➢ *The Older Adult Psychotherapy Treatment Planner* (Frazer, Hinrichsen, & Jongsma)

➢ *The School Counseling and School Social Work Treatment Planner* (Knapp, Jongsma, & Dimmitt)

➢ *The Crisis Counseling and Traumatic Events Treatment Planner* (Kolski, Jongsma, & Myer)

Finally, it is important to remember that the purpose of this series is to demonstrate the process of evidence-based psychotherapy treatment planning for common mental health problems. It is designed to be informational in nature, and does not intend to be a substitute for clinical training in the interventions discussed and demonstrated. In accordance with ethical guidelines, therapists should have competency in the services they deliver.

A

A Sample Evidence–Based Treatment Plan for Anorexia Nervosa

Primary Problem: Anorexia Nervosa

Behavioral Definitions:

1. Refusal to maintain body weight at or above a minimally normal weight for age and height (i.e., body weight less than 85% of that expected)
2. Intense fear of gaining weight or becoming fat, even though underweight
3. Persistent preoccupation with body image related to grossly inaccurate assessment of self as overweight
4. Undue influence of body weight or shape on self-evaluation
5. In post-menarcheal females, amenorrhea (i.e., the absence of at least three consecutive menstrual cycles)

Diagnosis: Anorexia Nervosa, Restricting Type (307.1)

Long-Term Goal:

1. Restore normal eating patterns, healthy weight maintenance, and a realistic appraisal of body size.

Objectives	Interventions
1. In a private session(s), have adolescent honestly describe the pattern of restricted eating from its start to the present.	1. Establish rapport with the client toward building a therapeutic alliance. 2. Assess the amount, type, and pattern of the client's food intake over the course of the disorder; assess perceived personal and interpersonal triggers and personal goals. 3. Assess the client for minimization and denial of the eating disorder behavior and related distorted thinking and self-perception of body image; assess motivation for change.
2. Describe any regular use of unhealthy weight control behaviors.	1. Assess for the presence of self-induced vomiting behavior by the client to purge himself/herself of calorie intake; monitor on an ongoing basis. 2. Assess for nonpurging compensatory behaviors by the client, such as misuse of laxatives, diuretics, enemas, or other medications; fasting; or excessive exercise; monitor on an ongoing basis.

(continued)

Objectives	Interventions
3. In a private session, parents describe their experiences and impressions of the client's anorexia from its start to the present.	1. Establish rapport with the parents toward building a therapeutic alliance. 2. Assess the parents' perceptions of the anorexia, including its nature, triggers, parental goals, and family strengths and weaknesses.
4. Complete psychological testing or objective questionnaires for assessing eating disorders.	1. Administer psychological instruments to the client designed to objectively assess eating disorders (e.g., Eating Inventory by Stunkard and Messick; Stirling Eating Disorder Scales by Williams and Power; or Eating Disorders Inventory-3 [EDI-3] by Garner); give the client feedback regarding the results of the assessment; readminister tests as needed to assess treatment outcome.
5. Cooperate with a complete medical evaluation.	1. Refer the client to a physician for a medical evaluation to assess current health status, including negative consequences of failure to maintain adequate body weight and overuse of compensatory behaviors; stay in close consultation with the physician as to the client's medical condition and needs.
6. Cooperate with a nutritional evaluation.	1. Refer the client to a nutritionist who is experienced in eating disorders for an assessment of nutritional rehabilitation; coordinate recommendations into the care plan.
7. Cooperate with admission to inpatient treatment, if indicated.	1. Refer the client for hospitalization, as necessary, if his/her weight loss becomes severe and physical health is jeopardized, or if he/she is severely depressed or suicidal.
8. Verbalize an understanding of the need, rationale, and goals of treatment.	1. Discuss a rationale for treatment that includes the seriousness of the disorder, the need for initial parental control over eating, and the coordination of medical, nutritional, and psychological care; overview the nature of the treatment and its goals.
9. Parents and adolescent with anorexia agree to participate in all three phases of family-based therapy of anorexia through approximately 20 sessions over 12 months.	1. Begin Phase 1 (sessions 1–10) of family-based treatment by confirming with the family their intent to participate and strictly adhere to the treatment plan, taking a history of the eating disorder, clarifying that the parents will be in charge of weight restoration of the client, establishing healthy weight goals, and asking the family to participate in the family meal in session; establish with the parents and a physician a minimum daily caloric intake for the client and focus them on meal planning; consult with physician and/or nutritionist if fluids and electrolytes need monitoring due to poor nutritional habits. 2. In Phase 2 (sessions 11–16), continue to closely monitor weight gain and physician/nutritionist reports regarding health status; gradually return control over eating decisions back to the adolescent as the acute starvation is resolved and portions consumed are nearing what is normally expected and weight gain in demonstrated. 3. In Phase 3 (sessions 17–20), review and reinforce progress and weight gain; focus on adolescent development issues; teach and rehearse problem-solving and relapse prevention skills.

B

Chapter Review Test Questions and Answers Explained

Chapter 1: What Are the Eating Disorders and Obesity?

1. Which of the following best differentiates bulimia nervosa (BN) from binge-eating disorder (BED)?

    A. BED is not associated with the compensatory behaviors aimed at preventing weight gain characteristic of BN.
    B. BN is not associated with the binge eating characteristic of BED.
    C. In BED, body weight is significantly lower than normal relative to BN.
    D. There are more attempts to diet in BN than in BED.

        A. *Correct*: Both BN and BED involve binging behavior, but only BN is associated with the compensatory behaviors, such as excessive exercise or self-induced vomiting, aimed at preventing weight gain.
        B. *Incorrect*: Binge eating is a diagnostic feature of both BED and BN.
        C. *Incorrect*: Body weight is not a diagnostic feature of BED or BN, although it is with anorexia nervosa. In terms of clinical presentation, patients with BED and BN are often overweight to varying degrees.
        D. *Incorrect*: Because of the absence of compensatory behaviors aimed at losing weight in BED, client histories are often characterized by attempt to lose weight through dieting.

2. True or False? Binge eating is characteristic of bulimia nervosa and binge-eating disorder, but is not seen in anorexia nervosa (AN).

    False.   Some patients who meet the diagnostic criteria for AN also engage in binge eating and purging. When this is the case, the *DSM-IV-TR* asks that the diagnosis specify this (i.e., "Anorexia Nervosa, Binge-Eating/Purging Type").

Chapter 2: What Are the Six Steps in Building a Treatment Plan?

1. As noted previously, some patients with eating disorders may use compensatory behaviors aimed at preventing weight gain, and some do not. Those who do may use purging types (e.g., self-induced vomiting), while others may not (e.g., excessive exercise). In which step of treatment planning would you record the particular expressions of the eating disorder for your individual client?

   A. Creating short-term objectives
   B. Describing the problem's manifestations
   C. Identifying the primary problem
   D. Selecting treatment interventions

      A. *Incorrect*: Expressions of the disorder, also referred to as manifestations, features, or symptoms, are described in Step 2 of treatment planning. They are not objectives for the client to achieve.
      B. *Correct*: Expressions of the disorder, also referred to as manifestations, features, or symptoms, are described in Step 2 of treatment planning.
      C. *Incorrect*: Expressions of the disorder, also referred to as manifestations, features, or symptoms, are described in Step 2 of treatment planning. They are expressions of the primary problem: the substance use disorder.
      D. *Incorrect*: Expressions of the disorder, also referred to as manifestations, features, or symptoms, are described in Step 2 of treatment planning. They are not interventions that the therapist will use to help the client achieve his or her objectives.

2. The statement "Learn and implement coping skills to resist urges to purge the body of food (i.e., to surf the urge)" is an example of a statement describing which of the following elements of a psychotherapy treatment plan?

   A. A primary problem
   B. A short-term objective
   C. A symptom manifestation
   D. A treatment intervention

      A. *Incorrect*: The primary problem (Step 1 in treatment planning) is the summary description, usually in diagnostic terms, of the client's primary problem.
      B. *Correct*: This is a short-term objective (Step 5 in treatment planning). It describes a desired action of the client that is likely to help him or her reach a treatment goal.

    C. *Incorrect*: Symptom manifestations (Step 2 in treatment planning) describe the client's particular expression (i.e., features or symptoms) of the primary problem.

    D. *Incorrect*: A treatment intervention (Step 6 in treatment planning) describes the therapist's actions designed to help the client achieve his or her short-term objectives.

Chapter 3: What Is the Brief History of the EST Movement?

1. Which statement best describes the process used to identify ESTs?

    A. Consumers of mental health services nominated therapies.

    B. Experts came to a consensus based on their experiences with the treatments.

    C. Researchers submitted their works.

    D. Task groups reviewed the literature using clearly defined selection criteria for ESTs.

        A. *Incorrect*: Mental health professionals selected ESTs.

        B. *Incorrect*: Expert consensus was not the method used to identify ESTs.

        C. *Incorrect*: Empirical works in the existing literature were reviewed to identify ESTs.

        D. *Correct*: Review groups consisting of mental health professionals selected ESTs based on predetermined criteria such as *well-established* and *probably efficacious*.

2. Based on the differences in their criteria, in which of the following ways are *well-established* treatments different from those classified as *probably efficacious*?

    A. Only *probably efficacious* allowed the use of single-case design experiments.

    B. Only *well-established* allowed studies comparing the treatment to a psychological placebo.

    C. Only *well-established* required demonstration by at least two different, independent investigators or investigating teams.

    D. Only *well-established* allowed studies comparing the treatment to a pill placebo.

        A. *Incorrect*: Both sets of criteria allowed use of single-subject designs. *Well-established* required a larger series than did *probably efficacious* (see II under Well-Established and III under Probably Efficacious).

        B. *Incorrect*: Studies using comparison to psychological placebos were acceptable in both sets of criteria (see IA under Well-Established and II under Probably Efficacious).

        C. *Correct*: One of the primary differences between treatments classified as *well-established* and those classified as *probably efficacious* is that *well-established* therapies have had their efficacy demonstrated by at least two different, independent investigators (see V under Well-Established).

D. *Incorrect*: Studies using comparison to pill placebos were acceptable in both sets of criteria (see IA under Well-Established and II under Probably Efficacious).

Chapter 4: What Are the Identified Empirically Supported Treatments for Substance Use Disorder?

1. According to APA's Division 12, The Society of Clinical Psychology, which of the following has met their criteria for a well-established psychological treatment for anorexia nervosa (AN)?

   A. Cognitive-behavioral therapy (CBT)
   B. Interpersonal therapy (IPT)
   C. Family-based treatment (FBT)
   D. Supportive psychotherapy (SP)

     A. *Incorrect*: The efficacy of CBT for AN has not met this level of evidence as defined by this organization. In addition, existing evidence supports it only as a post-hospitalization outpatient intervention for anorexia nervosa designed to prevent relapse once a patient has gained weight in the context of inpatient treatment.
     B. *Incorrect*: The efficacy of IPT for AN has not met this level of evidence as defined by this organization.
     C. *Correct*: FBT has recently met this organization's highest level of evidence based on recent randomized controlled trials (see reference section under "Empirical Support").
     D. *Incorrect*: The efficacy of SP for AN has not met this level of evidence as defined by this organization.

2. Which of the following is *not* one of the empirically supported treatments for bulimia nervosa (BN) cited by APA's Division 12, The Society of Clinical Psychology?

   A. Cognitive-behavioral therapy (CBT)
   B. Interpersonal therapy (IPT)
   C. Family-based treatment (FBT)
   D. Supportive psychotherapy (SP)

     A. *Incorrect*: CBT meets criteria for a well-established treatment as defined by this organization.
     B. *Incorrect*: IPT meets criteria for a well-established treatment as defined by this organization.

C. *Incorrect*: FBT meets criteria for a probably efficacious treatment as defined by this organization.

D. *Correct*: SP has not been identified as an empirically supported treatment for BN.

Chapter 5: How Do You Integrate ESTs Into Treatment Planning?

Assessment/Psychoeducation

1. At what point in therapy is psychoeducation conducted?

   A. At the end of therapy
   B. During the assessment phase
   C. During the initial treatment session
   D. Throughout therapy
      A. *Incorrect*: Although there may be some psychoeducation done at this phase of therapy, psychoeducation is conducted throughout therapy.
      B. *Incorrect*: Although there is commonly some psychoeducation done at assessment, psychoeducation is conducted throughout therapy.
      C. *Incorrect*: Although it is common for psychoeducation to be done early in therapy, it continues throughout.
      D. *Correct*: Psychoeducation permeates all phases of therapy.

Family–Based Treatment for Anorexia

1. Which of the following is *not* characteristic of the first phase of family-based treatment for anorexia nervosa?

   A. Control over eating is given to the adolescent patient.
   B. Parents are placed in charge of the nutritional rehabilitation and weight restoration of their adolescent child.
   C. The family eats some meals in therapy while the therapist assesses interactions.
   D. The seriousness of the disorder is conveyed.
      A. *Correct*: This is characteristic of Phase 2 of the therapy, after sufficient weight has been restored and the adolescent and parents meet certain criteria that support its feasibility.
      B. *Incorrect*: This is a requirement of Phase 1 of the therapy.
      C. *Incorrect*: This is a common practice in Phase 1 of the therapy.
      D. *Incorrect*: This is one of the first emphases of Phase 1 of the therapy.

Cognitive–Behavioral Therapy for Bulimia

1. Which of the following is a primary focus of cognitive-behavioral therapy (CBT) for bulimia nervosa (BN)?

A. How bulimia is an expression of a fixation from an earlier stage of development
B. How early attachment problems with primary caregivers have made the client vulnerable to bulimic acting out
C. How interpersonal issues such as disputes with parents and grief underlie the bulimia
D. How the current cycle of binging, purging, and concerns about body weight and shape operate in a cycle to maintain the disorder

    A. *Incorrect*: CBT is a present-focused treatment aimed at helping clients break the cycle of binging and purging. This description reflects a possible focus of psychoanalysis.

    B. *Incorrect*: CBT is a present-focused treatment aimed at helping clients break the cycle of binging and purging. This description reflects a possible focus of some psychodynamic therapies.

    C. *Incorrect*: CBT is a present-focused treatment aimed at helping clients break the cycle of binging and purging. This description is more consistent with the research-supported interpersonal therapy for bulimia.

    D. *Correct*: A primary aim of CBT is to help a client break the present cycle of binging and purging.

Interpersonal Therapy for Bulimia

1. Which of the following best characterizes an emphasis of the first phase of interpersonal therapy (IPT) for bulimia nervosa?

A. Assessing important past and present relationships
B. Addressing grief
C. Addressing role transitions
D. Training interpersonal skills

    A. *Correct*: A thorough assessment of interpersonal relationships, called the Interpersonal Inventory is conducted during the first phase of IPT.

    B. *Incorrect*: An intervention such as this is characteristic of Phase 2 of the therapy.

    C. *Incorrect*: An intervention such as this is characteristic of Phase 2 of the therapy.

    D. *Incorrect*: An intervention such as this is characteristic of Phase 2 of the therapy should clinically significant interpersonal deficits be evident.

Behavioral Weight Loss Treatments

1. LEARN is the well-studied version of behavioral weight loss treatments. For what does the acronym stand?

    A. Labor, Engage, Act, Ply, and Now

    B. Lifestyle, Exercise, Attitudes, Relationships, and Nutrition

    C. Listen, Examine, Analyze, Review, and Note

    D. Love, Endear, Adore, Relate, and Nap

        A. *Incorrect*: See B. This sounds like work.

        B. *Correct*: The acronym captures the major areas of intervention in the treatment program.

        C. *Incorrect*: See B. This sounds like analysis.

        D. *Incorrect*: See B. This sounds good.

Chapter 6: What Are Considerations for Relapse Prevention?

1. Sam and his therapist are talking about future situations that could challenge him and potentially set him back if he encounters one. They plan to review these encounters and develop a plan for coping with them in common sessions. Which consideration in relapse prevention is being conducted in the current session?

    A. Developing a coping card

    B. Distinguishing between a lapse and relapse

    C. Encouraging the routine use of skills learned in therapy

    D. Identifying high-risk situations for a lapse

        A. *Incorrect*: John may use a coping card to help him remember the skills learned in therapy that he will use to manage the high-risk situations being identified in this vignette.

        B. *Incorrect*: This is a psychoeducational intervention designed in part to help prevent misinterpretation of potentially manageable setbacks as an unmanageable relapse.

        C. *Incorrect*: John may use the skills learned in therapy to manage the high-risk situations being identified in this vignette.

        D. *Correct*: The vignette describes identifying high-risk situations for a lapse. John and his therapist will then review them and develop a plan for managing each. They may rehearse the plan in session and/or through between-session exercises.

STUDY PACKAGE
CONTINUING EDUCATION
CREDIT INFORMATION
Evidence-Based Treatment Planning for Eating Disorders and Obesity

Our goal is to provide you with current, accurate and practical information from the most experienced and knowledgeable speakers and authors.

Listed below are the continuing education credit(s) currently available for this self-study package. *Please note: Your state licensing board dictates whether self study is an acceptable form of continuing education. Please refer to your state rules and regulations.*

Counselors: CMI Education Institute, Inc. is an approved provider of the National Board of Certified Counselors, NBCC Provider #: 5637. We adhere to NBCC Continuing Education Guidelines. This self-study package qualifies for **3.25** contact hours.

Social Workers: CMI Education Institute, Inc., #1062, is approved as a provider for social work continuing education by the Association of Social Work Boards (ASWB), 400 South Ridge Parkway, Suite B, Culpeper VA 22701. www.aswb.org. CMI Education Institute, Inc. maintains responsibility for the program. Licensed Social Workers should contact their regulatory board to determine course approval. Social Workers will receive **3.25** (clinical) continuing education clock hours for completing this self-study package. Course Level: All Levels.

Marriage and Family Therapists: This activity consists of **3.25** hours of continuing education instruction. Credit requirements and approvals vary per state board regulations. Please save the course outline, the certificate of completion you receive from this self-study activity and contact your state board or organization to determine specific filing requirements.

Psychologists: CMI Education Institute, Inc. is approved by the American Psychological Association to sponsor continuing education for psychologists. CMI maintains responsibility for this program and its content. CMI is offering these self-study materials for **3.0** hours of continuing education credit.

Addiction Counselors: CMI Education Institute, Inc. is an approved provider of continuing education by the National Association of Alcoholism & Drug Abuse Counselors (NAADAC), provider #: 00131. This self-study package qualifies for **4.0** contact hours.

Nurses/Nurse Practitioners/Clinical Nurse Specialists: This activity meets the criteria for an American Nurses Credentialing Center (ANCC) Activity CMI Education Institute, Inc. is an approved sponsor by the American Psychological Association, which is recognized by the ANCC for behavioral health related activities.

This self-study activity qualifies for **3.0** contact hours.

Registered Dietitians & Dietetic Technicians, Registered: CMI Education Institute, Inc., #PE001, is a Continuing Professional Education (CPE) Accredited Provider with the Commission on Dietetic Registration (CDR) from June 1, 2012 through May 31, 2015. Registered dietitians (RDs) and dietetic technicians, registered (DTRs) will receive **3.0** continuing professional education units (CPEUs) for completion of these program/materials. Continuing Professional Education Provider Accreditation does not constitute endorsement by CDR of a provider, program, or materials. This program/material is designated as LEVEL 2.

Other Professions: This activity qualifies for **3.25** clock hours of instructional content as required by many national, state and local licensing boards and professional organizations. Retain your certificate of completion and contact your board or organization for specific filing requirements.

Procedures:

1. Review the materials (publication and DVD).

2. If seeking credit, complete the posttest/evaluation form:

   -Complete posttest/evaluation in entirety; including your email address for the most prompt receipt of your certificate of completion.

   -Upon completion, mail to the address listed on the form along with the CE fee stated on the test. Tests will not be processed without the CE fee included.

Completed posttests must be received 6 months from the date of purchase. Your completed posttest/evaluation will be graded. If you receive a passing score (70% and above), you will be emailed/faxed/mailed a certificate of successful completion with earned continuing education credits. (Please include your email address on the posttest/evaluation form for fastest response) If you do not pass the posttest, you will be sent a letter via email indicating areas of deficiency, and another posttest to complete. The posttest must be resubmitted and receive a passing grade before credit can be awarded. We will allow you to re-take as many times as necessary (with no additional fee) to receive a passing grade.

If you have any questions, please feel free to contact our customer service department at 1.800.844.8260.

CMI Education Institute

A Non-Profit Organization Connecting Knowledge with Need Since 1979

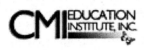 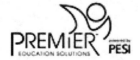

CMI Education PO BOX 1000 Eau Claire, WI 54702-1000

Education Institute

A Non-Profit Organization Connecting Knowledge with Need Since 1979

Evidence-Based Treatment Planning
for Eating Disorders and Obesity

Any persons interested in receiving credit may photocopy this form, complete and return with a payment of $15.00 per person CE fee. A certificate of successful completion will be sent to you. To receive your certificate sooner than two weeks, rush processing is available for a fee of $10. Please attach check or include credit card information below.

For office use only
Rcvd. _____
Graded _____
Cert. sent _____

Mail to: PESI, PO Box 1000, Eau Claire, WI 54702 or fax to PESI (800) 554-9775 (both sides)

CE Fee: $15: (Rush processing fee: $10)   **Total to be charged** _____

Credit Card #: _____ **Exp Date:** _____ **V-Code*:** _____
(*MC/VISA/Discover: last 3-digit # on signature panel on back of card.) (*American Express: 4-digit # above account # on face of card.)

Name (please print): _____ _____ _____
                                    LAST   FIRST   M.I.

Address: _____ Daytime Phone: _____

City: _____ State: _____ Zip Code: _____

Signature: _____ Email: _____

Date Completed: _____ Actual time (# of hours) taken to complete this offering: _____hours

Program Objectives After completing this publication, I have been able to achieve these objectives:

Explain the process and criteria for diagnosing eating disorders and obesity	Yes	No
List the six steps in building a clear psychotherapy treatment plan	Yes	No
Examine how empirically supported treatments for eating disorders and obesity have been identified	Yes	No
Illustrate objectives and treatment interventions consistent with those of identified empirically supported treatments for eating disorders and obesity	Yes	No
Explain how to construct a psychotherapy treatment plan and inform it with objectives and treatment interventions consistent with those identified empirically supported treatments for eating disorders and obesity	Yes	No
Identify common considerations in the prevention of relapse of eating disorders and obesity	Yes	No

Participant Profile:
1. Job Title: _____ Employment setting: _____

CMI Education
PO BOX 1000
Eau Claire, WI 54702-1000

ZNT044605   CE Release Date: 2/09/2012

Posttest Questions

1. According to psychiatric diagnostic classification systems, which of the following features is characteristic of anorexia nervosa, but not bulimia nervosa?
A. Concern about body shape and weight
B. Failure to maintain normal body weight
C. Tendency to binging eat
D. Use of purging to control weight

2. A 17-year-old female is brought to her pediatrician by her mother because of concerns that she is losing weight. The patient doesn't believe she has a problem and says that she actually is a little "chubby" in her face. She admits to occasionally binging on high-carbohydrate foods, feeling anxious and guilty, and then self-inducing vomiting to rid her of the calories. She is currently 20 percent below her normal expected body weight and shows evidence of amenorrhea. Which of the following diagnoses best captures this patient's features?
A. Anorexia Nervosa: Binge-eating/purging type
B. Anorexia Nervosa: Restricting type
C. Binge Eating Disorder
D. Bulimia Nervosa: Purging type

3. In reference to question 2, the patient's expression of her disorder, including her weight, binging, purging, and self-perception of being chubby despite having a low body weight would be recorded in which of the following steps in the treatment planning process discussed in this program?
A. Creating short-term objectives
B. Describing the problem's manifestations
C. Selecting therapeutic interventions
D. Specifying long-term goals

4. As discussed in this program, which of the following requirements was unique to APA Division 12's criteria for a well-established treatment, differentiating it from lesser levels of evidence such as probably efficacious?
A. Independent replication of efficacy studies was required.
B. Use of pill placebos in efficacy studies was required.
C. Use of psychological placebos in efficacy studies was required.
D. Use of random assignment in efficacy studies was required.

5. According to several reviewers of the psychotherapy outcome literature cited in this program, which of the following interventions has the highest level of evidence supporting its efficacy in the treatment of anorexia nervosa?
A. Behavioral weight loss programs
B. Cognitive behavioral therapy
C. Family-based therapy
D. Interpersonal therapy

6. According to this program, which of the following research-supported treatments for bulimia nervosa places strong emphasis on breaking the cycle of bingeing and purging using skills learned in therapy?
A. Behavioral weight loss programs
B. Cognitive behavioral therapy
C. Family-based therapy
D. Interpersonal therapy

7. According to this program, which of the following research-supported treatments for bulimia and binge eating disorder places a strong emphasis on understanding and resolving problems related to important past and/or present relationships in the patient's life?
A. Behavioral weight loss programs
B. Cognitive behavioral therapy
C. Family-based therapy
D. Interpersonal therapy

CMI Education
PO BOX 1000
Eau Claire, WI 54702-1000

Posttest Questions Continued

8. Which of the following characterizes phase one of family-based therapy for anorexia nervosa?
A. Siblings are placed in charge of the adolescent patient's re-feeding.
B. The adolescent patient is placed in charge of the re-feeding process.
C. The parents are placed in charge of the adolescent patient's re-feeding.
D. The therapist is placed in charge of the adolescent patient's re-feeding.

9. The LEARN program (i.e., Lifestyle, Exercise, Attitude, Relationship, and Nutrition) is an example of a behavioral weight loss program for obesity that has empirical support for its efficacy.
A. TRUE
B. FALSE

10. Which of the following best describes the approach to creating an evidence-based treatment plan for eating disorders that is recommended in this program?
A. The therapist conducts family-based therapy.
B. The therapist conducts interpersonal therapy.
C. The therapist incorporates into therapy the objectives and interventions consistent with research-supported treatments.
D. The therapist incorporates into therapy the use of an objective measure of the eating disorder to track treatment progress.

11. According to psychiatric diagnostic classification systems, which of the following features may be seen in bulimia nervosa, but not binge eating disorder?
A. A sense of lack of control while binging
B. Failure to maintain normal body weight
C. Tendency to binging eat
D. Use of purging to control weight

12. About 3 to 4 times a week, a 22-year-old female binge eats. During the binging she feels a lack of control over how much she is eating. Out of concern that she will gain weight, she misuses laxatives to purge her body of food. She feels guilty about her behavior, but is simultaneously concerned that others would not value her should she gain weight. Her BMI suggests that she is only slightly overweight currently. Which of the following diagnoses best captures this patient's features?
A. Anorexia Nervosa: Binge-eating/purging type
B. Anorexia Nervosa: Restricting type
C. Binge Eating Disorder
D. Bulimia Nervosa: Purging type

13. A therapist decides to include cognitive restructuring as part of the treatment plan for her client with bulimia nervosa. In which of the following steps in the treatment planning process should this be recorded?
A. Creating short-term objectives
B. Describing the problem's manifestations
C. Selecting therapeutic interventions
D. Specifying long-term goals

14. A treatment plan contains the sentence, "Use modeling and/or role-playing to train the client in assertiveness skills." In which of the following steps in the treatment planning process would this be recorded?
A. Creating short-term objectives
B. Describing the problem's manifestations
C. Selecting therapeutic interventions
D. Specifying long-term goals

Posttest Questions Continued

15. According to several reviewers of the psychotherapy outcome literature cited in this program, which of the following interventions has the highest level of evidence supporting its efficacy in the treatment of obesity?
A. Behavioral weight loss programs
B. Cognitive behavioral therapy
C. Family-based therapy
D. Interpersonal therapy

16. According to this program, which of the following research-supported treatments have the highest levels of evidence in the treatment of bulimia nervosa?
A. Behavioral weight loss programs and cognitive behavioral therapy
B. Cognitive behavioral therapy and interpersonal therapy
C. Family-based therapy and cognitive behavioral therapy
D. Interpersonal therapy and family-based therapy

17. According to this program, which of the following research-supported treatments has shown efficacy in the treatment of anorexia nervosa as well as for bulimia nervosa, albeit at different levels of evidence?
A. Behavioral weight loss programs
B. Family-based therapy
C. Interpersonal therapy
D. The LEARN program

18. Which of the following characterizes phase two of family-based therapy for anorexia nervosa?
A. Siblings are placed in charge of the adolescent patient's re-feeding.
B. The adolescent patient is placed in charge of the re-feeding process.
C. The parents are placed in charge of the adolescent patient's re-feeding.
D. The therapist is placed in charge of the adolescent patient's re-feeding.

19. According to this program, the American Psychological Association defines an evidence-based practice as the integration of the best available research with clinical expertise in the context of patient characteristics, culture, and preferences.
A. TRUE
B. FALSE

20. In identifying the evidence-based treatments cited in this program, the authors (i.e., Jongsma & Bruce) have used which of the following methods?
A. Establishing their own specific criteria for research support and citing those treatments that meet them
B. Identifying patterns of agreement across reviewers, review groups, and evidence-based practice guideline developers
C. Identifying treatments most preferred by patients/client
D. Identifying treatments most preferred by therapists

CMI Education
PO BOX 1000
Eau Claire, WI 54702-1000